Manual of Fast Track Recovery
for Colorectal Surgery

Nader Francis • Robin H. Kennedy
Olle Ljungqvist • Monty G. Mythen
Editors

Manual of Fast Track Recovery for Colorectal Surgery

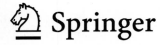 Springer

Editors
Nader Francis, MBChB, FRCS, PhD
Consultant Colorectal Surgeon
Department of Surgery
Yeovil District Hospital
Yeovil, Somerset
United Kingdom

Olle Ljungqvist, MD, PhD
Professor of Surgery
Department of Surgery
Örebro University Hospital
Örebro, Sweden

Robin H. Kennedy, MS, FRCS, MBBS
Consultant Colorectal Surgeon
St. Mark's Hospital
Harrow, United Kingdom

Monty G. Mythen, MBBS, FRCA,
FFICM, MD
Professor of Anaesthesia and Critical Care
Centre for Anaesthesia
University College of London
London, United Kingdom

ISBN 978-0-85729-952-9   e-ISBN 978-0-85729-953-6
DOI 10.1007/978-0-85729-953-6
Springer London Dordrecht Heidelberg New York

British Library Cataloguing in Publication Data
A catalogue record for this book is available from the British Library

Library of Congress Control Number: 2011944270

Springer is part of Springer Science+Business Media (www.springer.com)

Preface

Enhanced Recovery After Surgery (ERAS) has transformed perioperative care in modern surgical practice by emphasising the patients' optimal return to normal function after major surgery. The term ERAS was coined in 2001 by a group of academic clinicians (the ERAS Group) to replace the expression of 'Fast Track' surgery, and to emphasise the quality of the patients' recovery, rather than the speed of discharge. Subsequently, this group formed the ERAS Society for perioperative care (www.erassociety.org), which is facilitating the creation of this ERAS series, together with the British section of the society (ERAS-UK, www.enhancedrecoveryhub.org).

This book is long overdue. The most immediate didactic value resides in helping an entire multi-disciplinary ERAS team to understand the fundamental concepts and to deal with common problems in order to maintain success in ERAS. The manual hence focuses on practicalities, although it also contains chapters with more basic scientific content on the anaesthetic contribution, nutrition and metabolic response as well as audit and data collection for ERAS. The book thus fills an obvious need as a major bibliographical tool designed to facilitate the initial and ongoing practice of ERAS.

As ERAS originated in colorectal surgery, it is natural that the first manual in the series concerns this surgical discipline. However, much of the content will be equally applicable to other surgical specialties. As the ERAS methodology spreads, and more information and experience emerge, further manuals in the series will be published.

We are pleased to have several internationally renowned ERAS experts contributing to this book. The authors can be confident that there will be many grateful readers who will have gained a broader and scientific prospective on ERAS as a result of their efforts.

Olle Ljungqvist, Chairman

Ken Fearon, General Secretary

The Enhanced Recovery After Surgery (ERAS) Society for Perioperative Care.

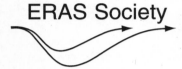

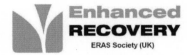

Foreword

Enhanced recovery programmes have the potential to transform the experience of care for large numbers of patients undergoing surgery. Pioneered in Denmark, enhanced recovery is now becoming firmly established across a range of disciplines within the UK, including colorectal, musculoskeletal, gynaecological and urological surgery. The benefits both to patients in terms of quicker recovery and to the health service in terms of efficient use of resources are clear cut.

Over the past 2 years I have had the pleasure and privilege of working with many champions and early adopters of enhanced recovery. I have been impressed by their commitment to spread the benefits of enhanced recovery as widely as possible and as quickly as possible. It is also clear that successful implementation requires close collaboration between surgeons, anaesthetists, nurses, dietitians and experts in rehabilitation.

Enhanced recovery involves multiple changes to practice both before, during and after surgery. I strongly commend this manual, which is authored by acknowledged experts in the field. They have set out the evidence base underlying enhanced recovery and combined this with practical advice on implementation.

Our challenge now is to ensure maximum benefit for patients within as short a timescale as is reasonably possible. This manual will help us all to meet this challenge.

Professor Sir Mike Richards
National Cancer Director

Contents

1   **Overview: Key Elements and the Impact
    of Enhanced Recovery Care** 1
    Kenneth C.H. Fearon

2   **Preoperative Optimisation and Conditioning
    of Expectations** 15
    John T. Jenkins and Jennie L. Burch

3   **The Metabolic Stress Response and Enhanced Recovery** 37
    Olle Ljungqvist

4   **Anaesthetic Contributions in Enhanced Recovery** 49
    Monty G. Mythen and Michael Scott

5   **Perioperative Fluid Management in Enhanced Recovery** 73
    Krishna K. Varadhan and Dileep N. Lobo

6   **Pain Control After Surgery** 95
    William J. Fawcett

7   **Colorectal Surgery and Enhanced Recovery** 111
    Matthew G. Tutton, N. Julian H. Sturt, and Alan F. Horgan

8   **Setting Up an Enhanced Recovery Programme** 131
    Fiona Carter and Robin H. Kennedy

9   **The Role of the Enhanced Recovery Facilitator** 143
    Jane P. Bradley Hendricks and Fiona Carter

10 **Success and Failure in Colorectal Enhanced Recovery** 159
    Nader Francis, Andrew Allison, and Jonathan Ockrim

11 **Data Collection and Audit** 171
    Jonas O.M. Nygren and Olle Ljungqvist

Index 177

Contributors

Andrew Allison Department of Surgery, Yeovil District Hospital,
Yeovil, Somerset, UK

Jennie L. Burch Department of Surgery, St. Mark's Hospital,
Harrow, Middlesex, UK

Fiona Carter Yeovil Academy, Yeovil District Hospital NHS Foundation Trust,
Yeovil, Somerset, UK

William J. Fawcett Department of Anaesthesia, Royal Surrey County Hospital
NHS Foundation Trust, Guildford, Surrey, UK

Kenneth C.H. Fearon Department of Surgical Oncology,
University of Edinburgh/Royal Infirmary, Edinburgh, UK

Nader Francis Department of Surgery, Yeovil District Hospital,
Yeovil, Somerset, UK

Jane P. Bradley Hendricks Department of General Surgery,
Colchester General Hospital, Colchester, Essex, UK

Alan F. Horgan Department of Surgery, Freeman Hospital, Newcastle, UK

John T. Jenkins Department of Surgery, St. Mark's Hospital,
London, Middlesex, UK

Robin H. Kennedy St. Mark's Hospital, Harrow, United Kingdom

Olle Ljungqvist Department of Surgery, Örebro University Hospital,
Örebro, Sweden

Dileep N. Lobo Nottingham Digestive Diseases Centre NIHR Biomedical
Research Unit, Nottingham University Hospitals, Queen's Medical Centre,
Nottingham, Notts, UK

Monty G. Mythen Centre for Anaesthesia, University College of London,
London, UK

Jonas O.M. Nygren Department of Surgery, Ersta Hospital and Karolinska Institutet at Danderyds Hospital, Stockholm, Sweden

Jonathan Ockrim Department of Surgery, Yeovil District Hospital, NHS Foundation Trust, Yeovil, Somerset, UK

Michael Scott Department of Anaesthetics and Intensive Care Medicine, Royal Surrey County NHS Foundation Trust, University of Surrey, Guildford, Surrey, UK

N. Julian H. Sturt Department of Surgery, Southend University Hospital NHS Trust, Westcliff-on-Sea, Essex, UK

Matthew G. Tutton ICENI unit, General Surgery, Colchester Hospital University NHS Foundation Trust, Colchester, Essex, UK

Krishna K. Varadhan Division of Gastrointestinal Surgery, Nottingham Digestive Diseases Centre NIHR Biomedical Research Unit, Nottingham University Hospitals, Queen's Medical Centre, Nottingham, Notts, UK

Chapter 1
Overview: Key Elements and the Impact of Enhanced Recovery Care

Kenneth C.H. Fearon

Introduction

Surgeons have had a long-standing interest in the immune and metabolic response to injury. Such interest has been spurred on by the recognition that modulation of these pathways might provide a route to reduce postoperative morbidity and mortality. Claude Bernard (France) first developed the concept of the milieu intérieur and Walter Cannon (USA) described the complex homeostatic responses involving the brain, nerves, heart, lungs, kidneys and spleen that work to maintain body constancy. Subsequently, Sir David Cuthbertson (UK) divided the metabolic response to injury into ebb, flow and recovery phases and quantified the amount and likely sources of protein breakdown following long bone fracture. Thereafter, individuals such as Francis Moore (USA) and Douglas Wilmore (USA) described in detail the response to injury in humans and methods of optimal nutritional and metabolic support. However, by the time of the second millennium the average length of hospital stay after colorectal abdominal surgery was still 10–15 days.

Against this background Henrik Kehlet (Denmark) started to question why patients undergoing elective abdominal surgery fail to go home sooner. He concluded that the key factors that keep a patient in hospital after uncomplicated major abdominal surgery include the need for parenteral analgesia (persistent pain), intravenous fluids (persistent gut dysfunction) and bed rest (persistent lack of mobility). These factors often overlap and interact to delay return of function. Obviously, postoperative complications will also prolong the time until recovery and ultimately length of stay. Kehlet went on to describe a clinical pathway to accelerate recovery after colonic resection based on a multimodal programme with optimal pain relief, stress reduction with regional anaesthesia, early enteral nutrition and early mobilisation – he demonstrated improvements in physical performance, pulmonary function, body

K.C.H. Fearon
Department of Surgical Oncology, University of Edinburgh/Royal Infirmary, Edinburgh, UK

N. Francis et al. (eds.), *Manual of Fast Track Recovery for Colorectal Surgery*,
Enhanced Recovery, DOI 10.1007/978-0-85729-953-6_1,
© Springer-Verlag London Limited 2012

composition and a marked reduction in length of stay [1–3]. A subsequent randomised trial using a similar protocol demonstrated a significant reduction in median length of stay from 7 to 3 days [4].

Since then many different groups have published variations on the nature of their optimal 'fast-track' or enhanced recovery programmes. For example, apparently similar outcomes can be achieved with [2–4] or without epidural anaesthesia/analgesia [5]. This suggests that it is the combination of each of the different elements of an enhanced recovery programme that goes to make an effective regimen rather than any single element on its own. At present, the evidence on which to base a multimodal programme is taken in isolation from traditional care pathways and little evidence is available concerning the importance of each element when considered within the context of an enhanced recovery pathway.

Principles of an ER Protocol

Conventional peri-operative metabolic care has accepted that a stress response to major surgery is inevitable. This concept has recently been challenged with the view that a substantial element of the stress response can be avoided with the appropriate application of modern anaesthetic, analgesic and metabolic support techniques. Conventional postoperative care has also emphasised prolonged rest for both the patient and their gastrointestinal tract. Similarly, this concept has recently been challenged. In the catabolic patient, medium-term functional decline will ensue if active steps are not taken to return the patient to full function as soon as possible. These two concepts have been combined to produce a new view of how surgical patients should be cared for (the ER protocol). Using a multidisciplinary team approach with a focus on stress reduction and promotion of return to function, an ER protocol aims to allow patients to recover more quickly from major surgery (Fig. 1.1), avoid medium-term sequelae of conventional postoperative care (e.g. decline in nutritional status and fatigue) and reduce healthcare costs by reducing hospital stay.

The move from traditional peri-operative care to an ER protocol is not straightforward. None of the elements within the ER protocol have been proven to be pivotal in

Fig. 1.1 Traditional peri-operative care often results in the patient being exposed to unnecessary metabolic/nutritional debilitation resulting in a prolonged recovery interval. A multimodal ER programme seeks to prevent such decline thereby allowing the patient to recover more quickly

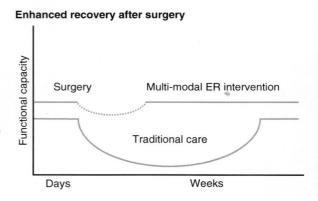

randomised trials. However, the ERAS group produced a comprehensive consensus of approximately 20 elements for patients undergoing colorectal resection in 2005 [6]. This protocol has been tested extensively, and a prospectively audited case-series including >1,000 patients was published in 2009 [7]. The protocol was recently updated [8] and the latter forms the basis for most of the recommendations in the present chapter.

To date, the most frequently used model for ER has been open colorectal resection. However, there is no doubt that the same principles can be applied successfully to other forms of major surgery (e.g. hepatic resection) [9]. Equally, the last 20 years has seen the revolution in laparoscopic surgery making a real impact on the rate at which patients recover from procedures such as cholecystectomy. At present the boundaries of laparoscopic surgery are being advanced into other domains such as colorectal resection. What is likely is that whether surgery is preformed by 'open' or laparoscopic means, if an ER protocol is not followed then the potential for the optimal recovery rate will not be achieved.

Key Elements of an ER Protocol

The elements of an ER protocol are diverse and varied (Fig. 1.2). The present chapter aims to cover a proportion of the key elements. Elements that are discussed in detail in subsequent chapters are not dealt with here.

In order to implement an ER protocol there must be an enthusiastic multidisciplinary team that works in a coordinated way (Table 1.1). Implementation is a radical and sometimes painful process and no member of the team should be focussed

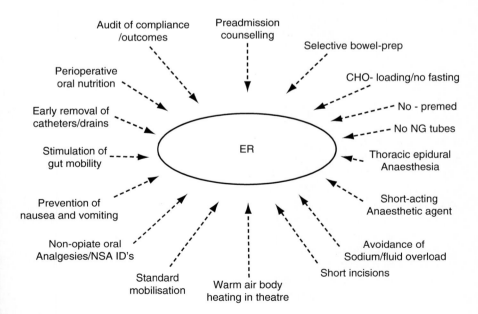

Fig. 1.2 Elements of an enhanced recovery (*ER*) protocol

Table 1.1 The members of the multidisciplinary team required to run a successful ER programme

Nurses
Dietitians
Physiotherapists
Occupational therapists
Pain team
Theatre staff
Anaesthetists
Surgeons
Hospital management
Audit team

on one single area of the patient's journey. Every member of the team should be trying to optimise outcome right from the first attendance at the outpatient clinic to the time of discharge home.

Preadmission Information and Counselling

Explicit preoperative patient information can facilitate postoperative recovery and pain control, particularly in patients who exhibit the most denial and highest levels of anxiety [10, 11]. A clear explanation of what is to happen during hospitalisation facilitates adherence to the care pathway and allows timely recovery and early discharge [12, 13]. Importantly, at this first encounter the patient should also be given a clear role with specific tasks to perform, including targets for food intake and oral nutritional supplements and targets for mobilisation, during the postoperative period [14, 15].

Preoperative Fasting and Metabolic Conditioning

Although fasting after midnight has been standard practice to avoid pulmonary aspiration in elective surgery, a review of recent studies has found no scientific support for this [16]. Equally, a recent Cochrane systematic review of 22 RCTs in adult patients provides robust evidence that reducing the preoperative fasting period for clear fluids to 2 h does not lead to an increase in complication rates [17]. Similar evidence is available for children undergoing surgery [18]. Several National Anaesthesia Societies now recommend intake of clear fluids up until 2 h before induction of anaesthesia and a 6 h fast for solid food and liquids containing fat or particulate material [19–21].

Patients should be in a metabolically fed state rather than fasted when they go to theatre. This can be achieved by provision of a clear carbohydrate-rich beverage before midnight and 2–3 h before surgery. This reduces preoperative thirst, hunger and anxiety [17, 22], and significantly reduces postoperative insulin resistance [23]. This also results in patients being in a more anabolic state with less postoperative nitrogen and protein losses [24, 25], better maintained lean body mass [26] and muscle strength [27]. Data from RCTs indicate enhanced recovery and shorter hospital stay from preoperative carbohydrate loading in colorectal surgery [28, 29].

Anaesthetic Protocols

The evidence to direct the choice of the optimal anaesthetic method for ER procedures is complex and controversial. However, it is rational to use short-acting agents (propofol, remifentanil) [30], thereby allowing proactive recovery to start on the day of surgery. Long-acting i.v. opioids (morphine, fentanyl) should be avoided. Short-acting inhalational anaesthesia is a reasonable alternative to total intravenous anaesthesia. There is no evidence that intraoperative epidural analgesia improves postoperative outcome in colorectal procedures, but its use reduces the dosage of general anaesthetic agents. Also, a mid-thoracic epidural activated before commencement of surgery blocks stress hormone release and attenuates postoperative insulin resistance [31]. For colonic surgery the epidural catheter is best placed at the mid-thoracic level (T7/8) to achieve both analgesia and sympathetic blockade preventing gut paralysis [32]. The catheter is sited in the awake patient to establish the effectiveness of the block. During surgery the block can be maintained by continuous infusion of local anaesthetic (e.g. bupivacaine 0.1–0.25% or ropivacaine 0.2%) plus a low-dose opiate (e.g. 2 µg/mL fentanyl or 0.5–1 µg/mL sufentanil) at 4–10 mL/h. Epidural opioids in small doses act in synergy with epidural local anaesthetics in providing analgesia [33], and without major systemic effects [34, 35]. Addition of adrenaline (1.5–2.0 µg/mL) to the thoracic epidural infusion can improve analgesia and decrease systemic opioid-related side effects [36].

Surgical Technique

A recent and comprehensive meta-analysis confirms that significant improvements in short-term outcomes are achievable by laparoscopy-assisted colonic resection as a single intervention [37]. Laparoscopic resection was associated with significant reductions in short-term wound morbidity as well as a significantly shorter time to first bowel movement and discharge from hospital.

The potential from combining laparoscopy with enhanced recovery care has only been evaluated in two small trials randomising patients to either laparoscopy-assisted or open surgery within an established, comprehensive enhanced recovery protocol [38, 39]. In the setting of a long-established and highly efficient enhanced recovery protocol, no further improvement in short-term outcome was seen by adding laparoscopy (median postoperative LOS of 2 days in both groups) [38]. The second study had longer hospitalisations, and here a reduction in postoperative LOS was seen in the laparoscopy-assisted group (3.5 vs. 6 days) [39]. Further investigation will hopefully more clearly evaluate the full potential of combining laparoscopy and enhanced recovery principles [40].

Surgical Incisions

There is evidence from some RCTs that transverse or curved incisions cause less pain and pulmonary dysfunction than vertical incisions following abdominal procedures [41, 42], while other trials have found no advantage of transverse incisions [43, 44]. It has also been shown that both right and left colonic resections can be performed through either type of incision [43, 45], and that there is no difference in outcome for left-sided colorectal procedures [45]. A recent Cochrane systematic review of RCTs comparing midline with transverse incisions for abdominal surgery confirms that although analgesic use and pulmonary compromise may be reduced with transverse or oblique incisions, this does not seem to be significant clinically as complication rates and recovery times are the same as with midline incisions [46]. The fact that some departments always use transverse or curved incision while other always use midline incisions provides circumstantial evidence that sufficient access to the surgical site can be obtained by either type of incision. However, it is clear that incision length affects patient recovery [47], and the choice of incision for abdominal surgery still remains the preference of the surgeon.

Multimodal Pain Relief

Several meta-analyses have shown that optimal analgesia is best achieved by continuous epidural local anaesthetic or local anaesthetic-opioid techniques for 2–3 days postoperatively [34, 48]. The advantage of epidural analgesia has also been demonstrated in laparoscopic surgery [49]. Analgesia based on intravenous opioids does not provide the same efficient analgesia [48] and has less beneficial physiological effects on surgical stress responses compared with epidural local anaesthetic techniques. Whilst it is possible to achieve almost the same pain scores with patient-controlled analgesia (PCA) at rest compared with epidural analgesia, this is done at the expense of the patient remaining sedated and in bed. RCTs have demonstrated that continuous epidural local anaesthetic techniques reduce pulmonary morbidity, but not other types of morbidity, hospital stay or convalescence [48, 50].

There are some concerns about the safety of epidural analgesia for colonic resection and anastomotic complications [48, 51, 52]. Perfusion of the splanchnic area, once epidural block has been established, is probably more closely associated with changes in mean arterial pressure than with changes in cardiac output [53]. Vasopressors should, therefore, be considered to improve colonic blood flow. Low-dose noradrenaline and dobutamine are probably not harmful for splanchnic perfusion [54–58]. The unanswered questions are the acceptable range of blood pressure in individual patients and the duration for which vasopressors should be used [51].

Once the epidural catheter is removed, the goal remains avoidance of opioids, thereby avoiding opioid-related side effects. NSAIDs have been shown to be opioid-sparing [59] and to provide efficient analgesia during this period after colon resection in large case series [2, 60].

Promoting Early Oral Intake

Postoperative ileus is a major cause of delayed discharge from hospital after abdominal surgery and its prevention is a key objective in enhanced recovery protocols. While no prokinetic agent currently available has been shown to be effective in attenuating or treating postoperative ileus, several other peri-operative interventions have been successful. Epidural analgesia, as compared with intravenous opioid analgesia, is highly efficient at preventing postoperative ileus [35, 48], provided it is mid-thoracic rather than low-thoracic or lumbar [32]. Fluid overloading during [61], and following [62], surgery has been demonstrated to significantly impair postoperative gastrointestinal function, and should be avoided. Oral magnesium oxide has been demonstrated to be effective in promoting postoperative bowel function in RCTs after abdominal hysterectomy [63] and hepatic resection [64], and in case series following colonic resection. Laparoscopy-assisted colonic resection also leads to faster return of bowel function as well as resumption of oral diet, as compared with open surgery [37]. In the USA, alvimopan was recently the first mu-opioid receptor antagonist to be approved for clinical use in postoperative ileus. This oral medication accelerates gastrointestinal recovery and reduces time to discharge in patients undergoing colon resection with postoperative intravenous opioid analgesia [65].

Other factors that impact on restoration of normal food intake include avoidance of routine nasogastric intubation [66], control of post-op nausea and vomiting, access to adequate normal food, access to oral nutritional supplements and integration of all of the above within the context of an enhanced recovery programme. When used in combination, early enteral feeding and epidural analgesia have been shown to result in almost complete abrogation of the metabolic response to injury with maintenance of energy and protein homeostasis [67]. This emphasises the importance of multimodal therapy in the maintenance of nutritional status following surgery.

Early Mobilisation

Bed rest not only increases insulin resistance and muscle loss but also decreases muscle strength, pulmonary function and tissue oxygenation [68]. There is also an increased risk of thromboembolism. In a randomised study, 3 months of a combination of aerobic and resistance training 5 times weekly, starting immediately after colorectal surgery, attenuated significantly the reduction in fatigue and lean body mass 7 days postoperatively [69, 70]. However, no improvement was found in body composition, nutritional intake or physiological function compared to the control group (relaxation training only) at day 30 or 90 after surgery. Effective pain relief using ambulatory thoracic epidural analgesia is a key adjuvant measure to encourage postoperative mobilisation. A prescheduled care plan should list daily goals for mobilisation, and a patient diary for out-of-bed activities is helpful. It is essential that the patient is nursed in an environment which encourages early mobilisation (food and television removed from bedroom) and one that maintains the patient's independence (ordinary ward/level 1 facility). The aim is for patients to be out of bed for 2 h on the day of surgery, and for 6 h a day until discharge.

Discharge Criteria

Patients can be discharged when they meet the following criteria:

Good pain control with oral analgesia
Taking solid food, no intravenous fluids
Independently mobile or same level as prior to admission
All of the above and willing to go home.

The discharge process starts at the preadmission counselling session when it is determined if the patient lives alone and has any special needs (e.g. transport, social support, etc). Problems that will delay discharge must be addressed at this time rather than once the patient has been admitted. It is clear that in most centres there is a delay between the time when the patient is recovered functionally and when they are actually discharged home [71] (Fig. 1.3). Minimising this delay requires optimal discharge planning.

Fig. 1.3 Minimising the delay between functional recovery and actual discharge. Will maximise the benefit of an ER programme in terms of length of stay

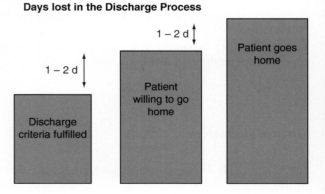

Days lost in the Discharge Process

1 – 2 d

Patient goes home

1 – 2 d

Patient willing to go home

Discharge criteria fulfilled

Outcomes

Enhanced recovery protocols have been developed to address the sequelae of the metabolic response to elective surgery and to accelerate recovery by attenuating the stress response so that the length of hospital stay and possibly the incidence of postoperative complications and mortality can be reduced, with the added benefits of reducing healthcare costs. These outcomes are difficult to address in small individual trials from single centres. A recent meta-analysis has, however, reported on six randomised trials of patients ($n=452$) undergoing major elective open colorectal surgery [72]. The number of individual ER elements used ranged from 4 to 12 with a mean of 9. The length of hospital stay was reduced by 2.5 days and complication rates were significantly reduced (relative risk [95% CI]: 0.53 [0.44, 0.64]). There were no statistically significant differences in readmission and mortality rates. Such evidence suggests that ER pathways do indeed reduce the length of stay and complication rates after major open colorectal surgery *without* compromising patient safety.

Evidence from the literature supports the view that an ER pathway seems to reduce the overall healthcare cost [73, 74]. From a health economics point of view, the data suggest that, with the decrease in complications and hospital stay and similar readmission rates, the cost of treatment per patient would be significantly lower for those treated within an ERAS pathway than those receiving traditional care, despite the need for dedicated staff to implement the pathway.

The determinants of outcome within an ER programme are important to know so that protocols can be used to maximum efficiency on the correct groups of patients. It is evident that a protocol is not enough to implement an ER programme and that compliance with the protocol both pre-op and post-op is vital if good results are to be obtained [71]. Compliance is a complex issue that requires audit of the process throughout the patient's journey, ongoing motivation from the team leaders, support from the hospital managers and regular/ongoing (re-) education of staff. Equally, it is evident that although good functional recovery may be obtained with experience and protocol compliance, the organisation of healthcare services to facilitate discharge into the community needs to be optimal if the delay between a patient's functional recovery and their actual discharge date is to be kept to a minimum.

Ultimately, outcomes are determined by the nature of the intervention and the pre-existing condition of the patient. In a large case-series of patients undergoing open colorectal resection ($n=1,035$) and managed within an ER programme [7] it was reported that independent predictors of delayed mobilisation were comorbidity (ASA grade III and IV) and age >80 years. Prolonged hospital stay was also related to comorbidity and advanced age but, in addition, the magnitude and technical difficulty of the surgery. ER programmes have developed considerably since first initiated by Kehlet in the 1980s. The individual elements that make up such programmes will continue to evolve. However, it would now appear that current programmes can indeed minimise the impact of surgery and its sequelae and that limiting factors which may dominate in the future will be related to pre-existing comorbidity and old age. Such issues constitute some of the real challenges for ER protocols in the future (Fig. 1.4).

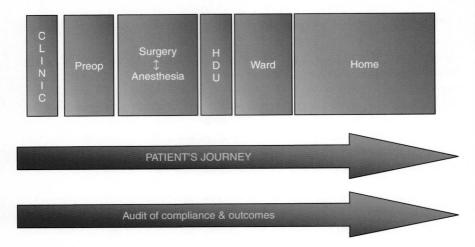

Fig. 1.4 Compliance within an ER programme requires that all staff integrate care across the patient's journey and that the entire process is subject to audit

References

1. Basse L, Raskov HH, Hjort Jakobsen D, Sonne E, Billesbolle P, Hendel HW, et al. Accelerated postoperative recovery programme after colonic resection improves physical performance, pulmonary function and body composition. Br J Surg. 2002;89(4):446–53.
2. Basse L, Hjort Jakobsen D, Billesbolle P, Werner M, Kehlet H. A clinical pathway to accelerate recovery after colonic resection. Ann Surg. 2000;232:51–7.
3. Basse L, Thorbol JE, Lossl K, Kehlet H. Colonic surgery with accelerated rehabilitation or conventional care. Dis Colon Rectum. 2004;47(3):271–7.
4. Anderson AD, McNaught CE, MacFie J, Tring I, Barker P, Mitchell CJ. Randomized clinical trial of multimodal optimization and standard perioperative surgical care. Br J Surg. 2003;90(12):1497–504.
5. Delaney CP, Fazio VW, Senagore AJ, Robinson B, Halverson AL, Remzi FH. 'Fast track' postoperative management protocol for patients with high co-morbidity undergoing complex abdominal and pelvic colorectal surgery. Br J Surg. 2001;88(11):1533–8.
6. Fearon KC, Ljungqvist O, von Meyenfeldt M, Revhaug A, Dejong CH, Lassen K, et al. Enhanced recovery after surgery: a consensus review of clinical care for patients undergoing colonic resection. Clin Nutr. 2005;24(3):466–77.
7. Hendry PO, Hausel J, Nygren J, Lassen K, Dejong CH, Ljungqvist O, et al. Enhanced Recovery After Surgery Study Group. Determinants of outcome after colorectal resection within an enhanced recovery programme. Br J Surg. 2009;96:197–205.
8. Lassen K, Soop M, Nygren J, Cox BW, Hendry PO, Spies C, et al. Consensus review of optimal peri-operative care in colorectal surgery. Arch Surg. 2009;144(10):961–9.
9. van Dam RM, Hendry PO, Coolsen MM, Bemelmans MH, Lassen K, Revhaug A, et al. Initial experience with a multimodal enhanced recovery programme in patients undergoing liver resection. Br J Surg. 2008;95:969–75.
10. Kiecolt-Glaser JK, Page GG, Marucha PT, MacCallum RC, Glaser R. Psychological influences on surgical recovery. Perspectives from psychoneuroimmunology. Am Psychol. 1998;53:1209–18.

11. Egbert LD, Battit G, Welch C, Bartlett M. Reduction of postoperative pain by encouragement and instruction of patients. A study of doctor-patient rapport. N Engl J Med. 1964;270: 825–7.

12. Halaszynski TM, Juda R, Silverman DG. Optimizing postoperative outcomes with efficient preoperative assessment and management. Crit Care Med. 2004;32:S76–86.

13. Forster AJ, Clark HD, Menard A, Dupuis N, Chernish R, Chandok N, et al. Effect of a nurse team coordinator on outcomes for hospitalized medicine patients. Am J Med. 2005;118: 1148–53.

14. Disbrow EA, Bennett HL, Owings JT. Effect of preoperative suggestion on postoperative gastrointestinal motility. West J Med. 1993;158:488–92.

15. Blay N, Donoghue J. The effect of pre-admission education on domiciliary recovery following laparoscopic cholecystectomy. Aust J Adv Nurs. 2005;22:14–9.

16. Ljungqvist O, Soreide E. Preoperative fasting. Br J Surg. 2003;90:400–6.

17. Brady M, Kinn S, Stuart P. Preoperative fasting for adults to prevent perioperative complications. Cochrane Database Syst Rev. 2003;4:CD004423.

18. Brady M, Kinn S, O'Rourke K, Randhawa N, Stuart P. Preoperative fasting for preventing perioperative complications in children. Cochrane Database Syst Rev. 2005;(2):CD005285.

19. Eriksson LI, Sandin R. Fasting guidelines in different countries. Acta Anaesthesiol Scand. 1996;40:971–4.

20. Soreide E, Eriksson LI, Hirlekar G, Eriksson H, Henneberg SW, Sandin R, et al. Pre-operative fasting guidelines: an update. Acta Anaesthesiol Scand. 2005;49:1041–7.

21. Practice guidelines for preoperative fasting and the use of pharmacologic agents to reduce the risk of pulmonary aspiration: application to healthy patients undergoing elective procedures: a report by the American Society of Anesthesiologist Task Force on Preoperative Fasting. Anesthesiology. 2001;90:1344–50.

22. Hausel J, Nygren J, Lagerkranser M, Hellstrom PM, Hammarqvist F, Almstrom C, et al. A carbohydrate-rich drink reduces preoperative discomfort in elective surgery patients. Anesth Analg. 2001;93:1344–50.

23. Nygren J. The metabolic effects of fasting and surgery. Best Pract Res Clin Anaesthesiol. 2006;20:429–38.

24. Crowe PJ, Dennison A, Royle GT. The effect of pre-operative glucose loading on postoperative nitrogen metabolism. Br J Surg. 1984;71:635–7.

25. Svanfeldt M, Thorell A, Hausel J, Soop M, Rooyackers O, Nygren J, et al. Randomized clinical trial of the effect of preoperative oral carbohydrate treatment on postoperative whole-body protein and glucose kinetics. Br J Surg. 2007;94:1342–50.

26. Yuill KA, Richardson RA, Davidson HIM, Garden OJ, Parks RW. The administration of an oral carbohydrate-containing fluid prior to major elective upper-gastrointestinal surgery preserves skeletal muscle mass postoperatively – a randomised clinical trial. Clin Nutr. 2005;24:32–7.

27. Henriksen MG, Hessov I, Dela F, Hansen HV, Haraldsted V, Rodt SA. Effects of preoperative oral carbohydrates and peptides on postoperative endocrine response, mobilization, nutrition and muscle function in abdominal surgery. Acta Anaesthesiol Scand. 2003;47:191–9.

28. Nygren J, Thorell A, Ljungqvist O. Preoperative oral carbohydrate nutrition: an update. Curr Opin Clin Nutr Metab Care. 2001;4:255–9.

29. Noblett SE, Snowden CP, Shenton BK, Horgan AF. Randomized clinical trial assessing the effect of Doppler-optimized fluid management on outcome after elective colorectal resection. Br J Surg. 2006;93:1069–76.

30. British national formulary 55. London: BMJ Group and RPS Publishing; 2008.

31. Uchida I, Asoh T, Shirasaka C, Tsuji H. Effect of epidural analgesia on postoperative insulin resistance as evaluated by insulin clamp technique. Br J Surg. 1988;75:557–62.

32. Miedema BW, Johnson JO. Methods for decreasing postoperative gut dysmotility. Lancet Oncol. 2003;4:365–72.

33. Liu S, Carpenter RL, Neal JM. Epidural anesthesia and analgesia. Their role in postoperative outcome. Anesthesiology. 1995;82:1474–506.

34. Block BM, Liu SS, Rowlingson AJ, Cowan AR, Cowan Jr JA, Wu CL. Efficacy of postoperative epidural analgesia: a meta-analysis. JAMA. 2003;290:2455–63.
35. Jorgensen H, Wetterslev J, Moiniche S, Dahl JB. Epidural local anaesthetics versus opioid-based analgesic regimens on postoperative gastrointestinal paralysis, PONV and pain after abdominal surgery. Cochrane Database Syst Rev. 2000;(4):CD001893.
36. Niemi G, Breivik H. The minimally effective concentration of adrenaline in a low-concentration thoracic epidural analgesic infusion of bupivacaine, fentanyl and adrenaline after major surgery. A randomized, double-blind, dose-finding study. Acta Anaesthesiol Scand. 2003;47:439–50.
37. Tjandra JJ, Chan MK. Systematic review on the short-term outcome of laparoscopic resection for colon and rectosigmoid cancer. Colorectal Dis. 2006;8:375–88.
38. Basse L, Jakobsen DH, Bardram L, Billesbolle P, Lund C, Mogensen T, et al. Functional recovery after open versus laparoscopic colonic resection: a randomized, blinded study. Ann Surg. 2005;241:416–23.
39. King PM, Blazeby JM, Ewings P, Franks PJ, Longman RJ, Kendrick AH, et al. Randomized clinical trial comparing laparoscopic and open surgery for colorectal cancer within an enhanced recovery programme. Br J Surg. 2006;93:300–8.
40. Wind J, Hofland J, Preckel B, Hollmann MW, Bossuyt PM, Gouma DJ, et al. Perioperative strategy in colonic surgery; LAparoscopy and/or FAst track multimodal management versus standard care (LAFA trial). BMC Surg. 2006;6:16.
41. Grantcharov TP, Rosenberg J. Vertical compared with transverse incisions in abdominal surgery. Eur J Surg. 2001;167:260–7.
42. Lindgren PG, Nordgren SR, Oresland T, Hulten L. Midline or transverse abdominal incision for right-sided colon cancer-a randomized trial. Colorectal Dis. 2001;3:46–50.
43. Brown SR, Goodfellow PJ, Adam IJ, Shorthouse AJ. A randomised controlled trial of transverse skin crease vs. vertical midline incision for right hemicolectomy. Tech Coloproctol. 2004;8:15–8.
44. Greenall MJ, Evans M, Pollock AV. Midline or transverse laparotomy? A random controlled clinical trial. Part II: Influence on postoperative pulmonary complications. Br J Surg. 1980;67:191–4.
45. Kam HM, Seow-Choen F, Peng XH, Eu KW, Tang CL, Heah SM, et al. Minilaparotomy left iliacfossa skin crease incision vs. midline incision for left-sided colorectal cancer. Tech Coloproctol. 2004;8:85–8.
46. Brown SR, Goodfellow PB. Transverse verses midline incisions for abdominal surgery. Cochrane Database Syst Rev. 2005;(4):CD005199.
47. O'Dwyer PJ, McGregor JR, McDermott EW, Murphy JJ, O'Higgins NJ. Patient recovery following cholecystectomy through a 6 cm or 15 cm transverse subcostal incision: a prospective randomized clinical trial. Postgrad Med J. 1992;68:817–9.
48. Marret E, Remy C, Bonnet F. Meta-analysis of epidural analgesia versus parenteral opioid analgesia after colorectal surgery. Br J Surg. 2007;94:665–73.
49. Zutshi M, Delaney CP, Senagore AJ, Mekhail N, Lewis B, Connor JT, et al. Randomized controlled trial comparing the controlled rehabilitation with early ambulation and diet pathway versus the controlled rehabilitation with early ambulation and diet with preemptive epidural anesthesia/analgesia after laparotomy and intestinal resection. Am J Surg. 2005;189:268–72.
50. Rigg JR, Jamrozik K, Myles PS, Silbert BS, Peyton PJ, Parsons RW, et al. Epidural anaesthesia and analgesia and outcome of major surgery: a randomised trial. Lancet. 2002;359:1276–82.
51. Low J, Johnston N, Morris C. Epidural analgesia: first do no harm. Anaesthesia. 2008; 63:1–3.
52. Fedder A, Dall R, Laurberg S, Rodt SA. Epidural anaesthesia with bupivacaine does not cause increased oedema in small gut anatomoses in pigs. Eur J Anaesthesiol. 2004;21:864–70.
53. Gould TH, Grace K, Thorne G, Thomas M. Effect of thoracic epidural anaesthesia on colonic blood flow. Br J Anaesth. 2002;89:446–51.
54. Woolsey CA, Coopersmith CM. Vasoactive drugs and the gut: is there anything new? Curr Opin Crit Care. 2006;12:155–9.

55. Thoren A, Elam M, Ricksten SE. Differential effects of dopamine, dopexamine, and dobutamine on jejunal mucosal perfusion early after cardiac surgery. Crit Care Med. 2000; 28:2338–43.
56. Seguin P, Laviolle B, Guinet P, Morel I, Malledant Y, Bellissant E. Dopexamine and norepinephrine versus epinephrine on gastric perfusion in patients with septic shock: a randomized study [NCT00134212]. Crit Care. 2006;10:R32.
57. Meier-Hellmann A, Sakka SG, Reinhart K. Catecholamines and splanchnic perfusion. Schweiz Med Wochenschr. 2000;130:1942–7.
58. Meier-Hellmann A, Reinhart K, Bredle DL, Sakka SG. Therapeutic options for the treatment of impaired gut function. J Am Soc Nephrol. 2001;12 Suppl 17:S65–9.
59. Cepeda MS, Carr DB, Miranda N, Diaz A, Silva C, Morales O. Comparison of morphine, ketorolac, and their combination for postoperative pain: results from a large, randomized, double-blind trial. Anesthesiology. 2005;103:1225–32.
60. Andersen J, Hjort-Jakobsen D, Christiansen PS, Kehlet H. Readmission rates after a planned hospital stay of 2 versus 3 days in fast-track colonic surgery. Br J Surg. 2007;94:890–3.
61. Nisanevich V, Felsenstein I, Almogy G, Weissman C, Einav S, Matot I. Effect of intraoperative fluid management on outcome after intraabdominal surgery. Anesthesiology. 2005;103: 25–32.
62. Lobo DN, Bostock KA, Neal KR, Perkins AC, Rowlands BJ, Allison SP. Effect of salt and water balance on recovery of gastrointestinal function after elective colonic resection: a randomised controlled trial. Lancet. 2002;359:1812–8.
63. Noblett SE, Watson DS, Huong H, Davison B, Hainsworth PJ, Horgan AF. Pre-operative oral carbohydrate loading in colorectal surgery: a randomized controlled trial. Colorectal Dis. 2006;8:563–9.
64. Hendry PO, van Dam RM, Bukkens SF, McKeown DW, Parks RW, Preston T, et al on behalf of ERAS Group. RCT to determine effect of post-operative laxation and its interaction into oral nutritional supplements within an ERAS protocol. Br J Surg. 2010;97:1198-1206
65. Delaney CP, Wolff BG, Viscusi ER, Senagore AJ, Fort JG, Du W, et al. Alvimopan, for postoperative ileus following bowel resection: a pooled analysis of phase III studies. Ann Surg. 2007;245:355–63.
66. Nelson R, Edwards S, Tse B. Prophylactic nasogastric decompression after abdominal surgery. Cochrane Database Syst Rev. 2007;(3):CD004929.
67. Soop M, Carlson GL, Hopkinson J, Clarke S, Thorell A, Nygren J, et al. Randomized clinical trial of the effects of immediate enteral nutrition on metabolic responses to major colorectal surgery in an enhanced recovery protocol. Br J Surg. 2004;91:1138–45.
68. Kehlet H, Wilmore DW. Multimodal strategies to improve surgical outcome. Am J Surg. 2002;183:630–41.
69. Houborg KB, Jensen MB, Hessov IB, Laurberg S. Little effect of physical training on body composition and nutritional intake following colorectal surgery – a randomised placebo-controlled trial. Eur J Clin Nutr. 2005;59:969–77.
70. Houborg KB, Jensen MB, Rasmussen P, Gandrup P, Schroll M, Laurberg S. Postoperative physical training following colorectal surgery: a randomised, placebo controlled study. Scand J Surg. 2006;95:17–22.
71. Maessen J, Dejong CH, Hausel J, Nygren J, Lassen K, Andersen J, et al. A protocol is not enough to implement an enhanced recovery programme for colorectal resection. Br J Surg. 2007;94(2):224–31.
72. Varadhan KK, Neal KR, Dejong CH, Fearon KC, Ljungqvist O, Lobo DN. The enhanced recovery after surgery (ERAS) pathway for patients undergoing major elective open colorectal surgery: a meta-analysis of randomized controlled trials. Clin Nutr. 2010;29:434–40.
73. Kariv Y, Delaney CP, Senagore AJ, Manilich EA, Hammel JP, Church JM, et al. Clinical outcomes and cost analysis of a 'fast track' postoperative care pathway for ileal pouch-anal anastomosis: a case control study. Dis Colon Rectum. 2007;50:137–46.
74. Kehlet H. Fast-track colonic surgery: status and perspectives. Recent Results Cancer Res. 2005;165:8–13.

Chapter 2
Preoperative Optimisation and Conditioning of Expectations

John T. Jenkins and Jennie L. Burch

Introduction

Enhanced recovery aims to reduce the systemic response to surgical stress and in doing so improve the quality and rapidity of a patient's recovery. It is a structured evidence-based process that encompasses the perioperative period of care and produces considerable reduction in postoperative complication rates and length of hospital stay [1–4]. The majority of patients undergoing elective colon and rectal surgery are suitable for this process. This chapter focuses on colorectal surgery but the principles are transferrable to many other surgical specialities. The chapter aims to cater to the needs of the multidisciplinary team, and a more detailed scientific explanation of some of the aspects covered in this chapter will be available from other sources. We explore the rationale for the preoperative optimisation and conditioning of expectations and describe how the multidisciplinary team can achieve this and how general practitioners can participate in the process.

The Rationale for Preoperative Optimisation and Conditioning of Expectations

For enhanced recovery to be successful it is essential that patients be adequately prepared for surgery and preoperative preparation is the first stage in this process. It sets the expectations of the patient and their family for planned surgery and emphasises how this can affect the patient. Pre-assessment requires liaison

J.T. Jenkins (✉)
Department of Surgery, St. Mark's Hospital, London, Middlesex, UK

J.L. Burch
Department of Surgery, St. Mark's Hospital, Harrow, Middlesex, UK

N. Francis et al. (eds.), *Manual of Fast Track Recovery for Colorectal Surgery*,   15
Enhanced Recovery, DOI 10.1007/978-0-85729-953-6_2,
© Springer-Verlag London Limited 2012

between primary and secondary care such that patient evaluation can identify medical and social factors that can be modified preoperatively, not only to reduce the effects of surgery upon the patient, but also ensure an efficient enhanced recovery process.

Pre-assessment Clinics

The pre-assessment, pre-admission or preoperative assessment clinic is the vehicle by which the early components of the enhanced recovery process are delivered and it allows for risk assessment and adjustment.

The key elements of the pre-assessment clinic are:

- *Full* assessment and clinical examination with anaesthetic consultation shortly after a decision to operate has been made.
- The patient has the maximum opportunity to optimise fitness for surgery and anaesthesia.
- Expectations are conditioned; the patient fully understands the proposed operation and is made ready to proceed.
- Staff identify and co-ordinate all essential resources and discharge requirements.
- Suitable admission *and discharge dates are agreed.*

This process is delivered by a specifically trained nursing team in close liaison with junior and senior surgical and anaesthesia staff and, where necessary, enterostomal therapists, occupational therapist, dietician and physiotherapist along with the patient's general practitioner. The aim is to assess the patient's fitness for anaesthesia and surgery and ideally, this interaction should be approximately 4 weeks before elective surgery, however, the nature of many colorectal cancer cases is such that this time frame is often a luxury owing to specified treatment time targets [5]. Employing the pre-assessment process means that cancellation owing to ill health or failure to attend can be avoided and same day admission and early discharge are more likely, producing improvements in the efficiency of a patient's care [6].

Treating Co-morbidity Before Surgery

A large population of high-risk general surgical patients exists, accounting for approximately 13% of all surgical admissions but more than 80% of postoperative deaths [7]. Successive NCEPOD reports indicate that most deaths occur in older patients who undergo major surgery and have severe co-existing disease with mortality rates between 5% and 25% [8].

Complications within 30 days in postoperative surgical patients have been found to be an important determinant of long-term survival and to be of a greater influence in some reports than preoperative co-morbidity and intraoperative adverse events. Avoiding or reducing complications is therefore of paramount importance. Detecting and modifying co-morbidities before an operation is central to the early stage of enhanced recovery and allows for a reduction in morbidity and in the need for more complex supportive care, such as intensive care [6]. Preoperative assessment allows realistic evaluation of the risk of surgical intervention and gives an opportunity to manage the risk to an individual patient by making modifications to improve the patient's general condition and organ function [9]. Understanding and quantifying the risk of perioperative complications and determining the likely type of complications are therefore required. These include cardiopulmonary morbidity and cardiac adverse events, postoperative gut dysfunction, surgical site infection, blood transfusion and the requirement for intensive care or high dependency care and readmission. Central to pre-assessment is optimisation through the determination of cardiovascular risk, nutrition, correction of anaemia and multiple other medical conditions.

Specific Examples

Cardiovascular Risk

The cardiovascular management of high-risk surgical patients is of particular importance and a large body of evidence now exists that can guide the clinician in delivering optimal care. The ACC/AHA Task Force Guidelines provide appropriate evidence-based guidance and are quoted throughout this chapter [10].

Major abdominal surgery is associated with a marked inflammatory response with an associated rise in tissue oxygen requirements that enforces a rise in the cardiac output. This response is related to the magnitude of tissue injury and surgical invasion and is associated with an elevation in heart rate and blood pressure with a neuroendocrine and thrombosis/fibrinolysis system response that predisposes high-risk patients to acute coronary events/syndrome, ischaemia and heart failure. The incidence of significant cardiovascular adverse events in a population undergoing noncardiac surgery such as the colorectal surgery population is approximately 1–2% and multiple risk factors have been associated. [7] These adverse events include cardiac arrest, non-ST elevation myocardial infarction (MI), Q-wave MI and new cardiac arrythmias. A patient's condition preoperatively, presence of co-morbidities [e.g., ischaemic heart disease (IHD), left ventricular failure (LVF)], pulmonary, renal disease and diabetes and the magnitude, duration and type of surgery will impact upon the likelihood of cardiovascular morbidity [7, 10, 11]. High-risk patients are those who are unable to spontaneously elevate their cardiac output to the required level. This at-risk group can be identified based upon clinical assessment and are likely to benefit from optimisation both preoperatively and intraoperatively.

The literature on cardiac adverse events has evolved from prediction to optimisation through intervention. The risk factors found to be independent predictors of outcome differ between analyses, and some traditional medical risk factors are believed to be less relevant today as the medical management of these conditions has improved, for example some of the risk factors identified in the Goldman criteria are no longer independent predictors on some more recent analyses, e.g., diabetes and chronic renal failure. Recent risk factors include age; congestive cardiac failure (CCF); body mass index (BMI) > 30; emergency surgery; previous cardiac intervention; cardiovascular disease (CVD); hypertension; duration of surgery; blood transfusion units; obesity has been previously found to be a predictor of coronary artery disease but more recent analyses find that an elevated BMI is an independent predictor of perioperative adverse cardiac events [7].

Though laparoscopy yields multiple short-term benefits for recovery, the advantages in patients with significant cardiac dysfunction have not been established. Therefore, cardiac risk in patients with heart failure is not diminished in patients undergoing laparoscopy compared with open surgery, and both should be evaluated in the same way [11].

Assessing Cardiac Risk and Need for Cardiology Assessment

Advances in preoperative risk assessment have reduced perioperative cardiovascular morbidity and rely on a complete history and physical examination to identify patients who have cardiovascular risks that may have previously been undocumented. Where a patient's history yields active cardiac conditions such as acute coronary syndrome, unstable angina, recent MI, decompensated heart failure, significant arrythmias or severe valvular disease, then elective colorectal surgery should be postponed until modifications are made in liaison with a cardiologist and the patient's general practitioner.

It is recommended that clinical risk indices be used for postoperative risk stratification [11]. During the last 30 years, several risk indices have been developed, based on multivariate analyses of observational data, which examine the association between clinical characteristics and perioperative cardiac mortality and morbidity [11–13]. These indices assist in the assessment of preoperative cardiac risk based upon the presence of defined clinical risk factors and the number of these risk factors allows triage to further assessment. The Lee index is a modification of the original Goldman index and currently regarded as the most informative cardiac risk prediction index for non-cardiac surgery, though it has some shortcomings [12]. The risk factors identified include 'high-risk surgery'; prior MI (according to the universal definition of MI); heart failure; stroke/transient ischaemic attack (TIA); renal dysfunction (serum creatinine >170 μmol/L or 2 mg/dL or a creatinine clearance of <60 mL/min); diabetes mellitus (DM) requiring insulin therapy. All factors contribute equally to the index (with 1 point each), with major cardiac complications estimated to be 0.4%, 0.9%, 7% and 11% in patients with an index score of 0, 1, 2 and 3 points, respectively. The index has a high capability for discriminating between

Table 2.1 Cardiac risk factors

Clinical factors	'Erasmus' index
Definitions in text	
Age	Y
IHD [Angina/IHD]	Y
Heart failure	Y
Stroke/TIA	Y
DM (on insulin)	Y
Renal dysfunction/Haemodialysis	Y
Surgical risk group	High, intermediate, low group

Note: Derived from a retrospective analysis of the Lee index from the administrative database of the Erasmus Medical Centre in Rotterdam, Netherlands, stratified by non-cardiac surgical procedure type. High-risk: [>5%, 30-day risk of cardiac death or MI] – e.g., aortic or vascular surgery; Intermediate [1–5% risk] – e.g., abdominal, head and neck, neurological, orthopaedic, transplant, urology, major; Low-risk [<1% risk] – e.g., breast, endocrine, gynaecological, urology, minor

patients who do and do not sustain a major cardiac event [11]. Modification with the refinement of the addition of a more detailed description of the type of surgery and age increases the prognostic value of the subsequent 'Erasmus' model for perioperative cardiac events (Table 2.1) [13].

'Functional capacity' is a measure of how well a patient is able to perform a spectrum of activities, an integral component of the preoperative evaluation of the cardiac risk patient for non-cardiac surgery and can be ascertained based upon a structured history [14]. For example, a patient's capacity to climb stairs has been found to have perioperative prognostic importance and can predict survival after lung resection and is associated with complications after major non-cardiac surgery [15–17]. After thoracic surgery, a poor functional capacity has been associated with an increased mortality. By making this assessment we can decide on the need for further investigation. There will be patients who are classified as high risk owing to age or coronary artery disease yet are asymptomatic and run for 30 min a day. Such a patient is unlikely to require further cardiac investigation and management will rarely be changed based on the results of any cardiovascular testing. In contrast, there will be patients who are sedentary with no recorded history of cardiovascular disease but are only able to manage to climb only a flight of stairs before the onset of symptoms. This group will require further cardiac evaluation.

Examples of activities are presented in Table 2.2 and determining functional capacity may prevent unnecessary cardiac evaluation and inefficient resource usage. One metabolic equivalent of task (MET) is the effort required whilst reading this chapter sitting. One MET represents the resting oxygen consumption of an adult (approximately 3.5 mL/kg/min) [18]. To some purist physiologists, the definition of MET is misinterpreted, however, a discussion on this aspect is beyond the scope of this chapter [19]. Nevertheless, the concept is helpful in assessing a patient's fitness for surgery.

Although assessment of functional capacity is useful in identifying patients with good or excellent capacity, where prognosis will be excellent even in the presence

Table 2.2 Functional capacity

MET	Activity	Capacity
<4 METS	– Unable to walk ≥ 2 blocks on level ground without stopping due to symptoms – Eating, dressing, toileting, walking indoors, light housework	Poor
>4 METS	– Climbing ≥ 1 flight of stairs without stopping – Walking up hill ≥ 1–2 blocks – Scrubbing floors – Moving furniture – Golf, bowling, dancing or tennis – Running short distance	Moderate/excellent [Excellent: >10 METS, Good: 7–10 METS, Moderate: 4–6 METS]

of stable IHD or other risk factors, its use in predicting survival after major non-cardiac surgery in those with a reduced functional capacity is less effective [11]. For example, as mentioned above, thoracic surgery outcome is strongly related to functional capacity, potentially reflecting the importance of lung function to functional capacity, however, this association has not been convincingly replicated with other non-cardiac surgeries and age has been found to be more predictive of a poorer outcome [17]. Therefore using functional capacity evaluation prior to surgery, measured by the ability to climb two flights of stairs or run for a short distance indicates a good functional capacity. On the other hand, when functional capacity is poor or unknown, it will be the presence and number of clinical risk factors suggested above in relation to the risk of surgery that will determine the preoperative risk stratification, assessment and perioperative management.

Other measures of risk have been assessed. For instance, how a patient performs under actual physical exertion has been tested [20, 21]. This has been termed cardiopulmonary exercise testing (CPEX or CPET) and to date is only available in a few centres in the UK. It has been employed to determine perioperative aerobic capacity and is reported in terms of the anaerobic threshold (AT). AT is the oxygen uptake at which anaerobic adenosine triphosphate (ATP) synthesis starts to supplement aerobic ATP synthesis. During gas exchange, it is the point at which the slope of CO_2 production increases more than the oxygen uptake. It is assumed that myocardial ischaemia develops at or above the AT, meaning that early ischaemia is associated with a lower AT and hence mortality, although non-cardiac and non-respiratory factors such as skeletal muscle function and physical training can underestimate aerobic metabolic activity. In simple terms, where an earlier switch from aerobic to anaerobic metabolism is required, poorer fitness is identified and a poorer outcome more likely.

A patient with a low AT is likely to benefit from more intensive perioperative care and risk modification [21]. For example, AT values of >11 mL/min/kg have a perioperative mortality of <1% and are unlikely to need higher level care; AT values ≤ 11 mL/min/kg have a perioperative mortality of 18% and should be considered for either intensive recovery, post-anaesthesia care unit (PACU), high-dependency unit

(HDU) or intensive care unit (ICU); AT <8 mL/min/kg have a perioperative mortality of 50% and should be considered and prepared for an extended stay in the ICU.

The real benefits of CPET in colorectal surgery are still unclear at the time of writing and whilst there may be a role in stratifying risk for the level of perioperative care, whether it changes clinical decision-making more than existing parameters is unclear. Therefore the role of CPET in preoperative risk assessment is yet to be established and CPET should not be considered to be a substitute for other forms of testing in routine practice.

What Investigations Should Be Considered?

The most suitable investigations in at-risk individuals are based upon clinical risk stratification assessed upon history, examination and determination of functional capacity as emphasised above (Table 2.3). Directed non-invasive investigation of patients with coronary artery disease and heart failure should only be considered where the results may effect a change in a patient's management, and therapy should only be changed where it will improve a patient outcome [10, 11]. These decisions are likely to be at the discretion of both anaesthetist and cardiologist and local preferences may vary.

12 Lead Resting ECG

Though the ideal time preoperatively to perform an electrocardiogram (ECG) is unclear, ideally it should be performed within 30 days of planned colorectal surgery and is indicated when patients are to undergo intermediate or major colorectal surgery and have at least one clinical risk factor such as ischaemic heart disease or an established history of coronary heart disease (CHD), peripheral arterial disease or cerebrovascular disease [10, 11].

Non-invasive Stress Testing

Echocardiography can be used to provide information on left ventricular (LV) function. Where a patient has breathlessness of unknown origin or has a history of current or prior heart failure with worsening breathlessness or any other change clinically, then echocardiography should be considered, particularly if an assessment has not been made within the preceding 12 months. In the setting of a known cardiomyopathy, if a patient has remained clinically stable then reassessing LV function would not be regarded as necessary [10, 11].

Echocardiography may be supplemented by pharmacological cardiac manipulation as in a dobutamine stress echocardiograpy (DSE). Non-invasive stress testing using techniques such as DSE are employed in patients with at least one to two clinical risk factors associated with a poor functional capacity (i.e. <4 METS) who are to undergo major colorectal surgery. DSE uses pharmacological manipulation

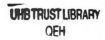

Table 2.3 Stepwise perioperative cardiac risk evaluation and management

	Step	Categories	Action	Management
Step 1	Assess for active cardiac conditions	Unstable angina Acute heart failure Significant cardiac arrythmia Symptomatic valvular heart disease Recent MI	*Postpone surgery* if active condition present Cardiology and Anaesthesia opinion Otherwise Step 2	Surgery after investigation and treatment
Step 2	Assess risk of surgical procedure	Low risk Intermediate and high risk	*Proceed with surgery* Move to Step 3 Assess functional capacity and clinical risk factors	
Step 3	Assess functional capacity	>4 METS and no symptoms Poor < 4 METS or unknown	*Proceed with surgery* Move to Step 4 Assess clinical risk factors Consider CPEX where available	
Step 4	Clinical risk factors	3 or more risk factors	Cardiology and Anaesthesia opinion: Stress testing [DSE] if will modify management	Optimise medical therapy and heart rate control before proceeding with surgery
		1 or 2 risk factors	Cardiology and Anaesthesia opinion: Stress testing [DSE] if will modify management Stress testing results	Optimise medical therapy and heart rate control before proceeding with surgery
		For no, mild or moderate stress-induced ischaemia, a statin and low-dose beta-blocker therapy are considered before surgery. For extensive stress-induced ischaemia, management is individualised and may employ optimal medical therapy, angioplasty, [drug-eluting] stenting or CABG.		
		No risk factors	*Proceed with surgery*	
Step 5	Surgery			

with increasing doses of supratherapeutic dobutamine that increases cardiac muscle contractility and the heart rate, which can be assessed by cardiac ultrasonography. It aims to identify significant coronary artery disease by identifying regional wall motion abnormalities within the distribution of the affected vessels [10, 11].

Cardiovascular risk in high-risk individuals may be minimised by coronary revascularisation where a large ischaemic burden is identified preoperatively, and/or by pharmacological intervention (e.g., beta blockers can reduce cardiac events/non-fatal MI and all-cause mortality), modifications to anaesthesia (e.g., neuraxial blockade, postoperative analgesia) and perioperative monitoring techniques.

Pulmonary Risk

Patients with co-existing pulmonary disease represent a group at higher risk of peri-operative morbidity, particularly pulmonary complications and mortality. Any condition causing impairment of lung function is culpable and includes chronic obstructive pulmonary disease (COPD), asthma, acute respiratory tract infections, interstitial lung disease and cystic fibrosis. One in ten patients is likely to have COPD and this is a major cause of morbidity and mortality [22]. Smokers are also at increased risk of pulmonary morbidity and the merits of even short-term smoking cessation a few weeks prior to surgery can be emphasised at the pre-assessment clinic. Emphasising the importance of postoperative mobilisation in the pre-assessment clinic encourages measures to prevent atelectasis. Other actions that a patient may participate in include deep breathing and incentive spirometry exercises. There is good evidence that these lung expansion interventions can reduce pulmonary risks in the perioperative period.

In general, if significant pulmonary disease is suspected based upon history or physical examination and determination of functional capacity then response to bronchodilators and the evaluation for the presence of carbon dioxide retention through arterial blood gas analysis may be justified. If there is evidence of infection, appropriate antibiotics are critical, and steroids and bronchodilators may need to be considered. Close liaison with a patient's general practitioner may facilitate this process.

Rarely, cardiac assessment may be required with pulmonary conditions for instance COPD and pulmonary arterial hypertension.

Anaemia

A large proportion of patients undergoing elective surgery for colorectal cancer are anaemic and iron deficient at the time of diagnosis. In the pre-assessment clinic it should established which type of anaemia is present and a full blood count (FBC) should be checked. Where other forms of anaemia are present then these should be managed according to appropriate local guidelines; however most patients are likely to have iron deficiency anaemia in the colorectal cancer group. It is recommended that elective surgery patients should receive a haemoglobin (Hb) determination a minimum of 30 days before the scheduled surgical procedure, however, this may not be feasible in the UK given colorectal treatment target times [23].

The need for blood transfusion may indicate a high-risk situation and in cardiac surgery the need for blood transfusion is an independent risk factor for mortality.

Mild anaemia is associated with a more advanced disease stage and is associated with a higher mortality, morbidity and length of hospital stay [24]. Unsurprisingly, some studies identify that a low preoperative haematocrit and haemoglobin level is an independent risk factor for blood transfusion [25] with transfusion rates of between 10% and 30% in the literature [26]. Blood transfusion, other than being an expensive and a limited resource, is associated with potentially serious complications, such as transfusion reactions and transmission of viral infection; is well recognised to be associated with higher postoperative systemic infection rates; and is also associated with a higher colorectal cancer recurrence rate with a dose-related increase in the odds of recurrence by 30% with every additional two units of blood that are transfused [26]. In addition, autologous transfusion (following self-donation) does not alter prognosis or decrease cancer recurrence risk when compared to allogeneic transfusion. Moreover, a theoretical risk of autologous transfusion is the reintroduction of tumour cells that may impair cancer outcome [27]. Transfusion also has the unwanted effect of immunosuppression and may alter outcomes owing to reduced tumour surveillance. It affects the immune system and on a cellular level seems to be associated with decreased T-cell-mediated immunity, induction enhancement of the acute inflammatory response and increased cytokine production. Leukocyte reduction of transfused blood neither changes recurrence rates nor survival in transfused colorectal cancer patients [28].

Blood transfusion and intense surgical stress might synergistically affect the long-term progress after curative resection of colorectal cancer and therefore avoiding transfusion where possible appears to be a sensible solution. Strategies in patients with anaemia are therefore centred upon increasing haemoglobin levels preoperatively without resorting to blood transfusion and restricting intraoperative surgical blood loss to an absolute minimum.

Debate exists regarding the threshold level of haemoglobin for intervention without transfusion and what the target level should be prior to surgery. A haemoglobin level of below 10 g/dL is often regarded as the minimum threshold for intervention but is likely to evolve as further evidence is published. There is also debate around the threshold for blood transfusion. Practice guidelines from the American Society of Anesthesiology suggest transfusion at a level of 6 g/dL but not at 10 g/dL [29]. In a patient within the range 6–10 g/dL, decisions therefore need to be taken based on individual circumstances (e.g., co-morbidity, organ ischaemia, intravascular volume, ongoing bleeding, risks of inadequate oxygenation).

Options to treat anaemia preoperatively to avoid transfusion include oral and intravenous iron supplements, with or without erythropoietin stimulation [30–33]. These agents have been submitted to study in randomised clinical trials in the correction of perioperative anaemia in an attempt to reduce allogeneic blood transfusion and the consequences above.

In colorectal cancer, Lidder found that 'oral ferrous sulphate given preoperatively in patients undergoing colorectal surgery offers a simple, inexpensive method of reducing blood transfusions' and improved the haemoglobin and ferritin levels [30]. Other groups have identified this benefit in non-randomised studies and have suggested that supplementation for at least 2 weeks prior to surgery is required [34]. Oral iron therapy is cheap but there are a number of caveats to its use. Patients already taking a variety of tablet and capsule medications may find the addition of oral iron a burden. Poor compliance, intolerance, duration of treatment, poor (unpredictable) response, continuing blood loss and anaemia of chronic disease (associated with inflammation and surgery) also restrict the appropriateness of oral iron therapy. Intravenous iron in some studies is felt to be more convenient and achieves target Hb levels and repletes iron stores more quickly but its role in colorectal cancer surgery has been less convincing to date.

A consensus statement published on the role of intravenous iron in perioperative management by Beris concluded that currently recommendations can be made for use in orthopaedic surgery and that more evidence is needed for surgery in other specialities such as colorectal surgery [35]. However, intravenous iron has been shown to be more effective than oral iron in post-partum anaemia, resulting in a more rapid rise and sustained Hb levels [36].

Erythropoietin levels are reduced in patients with cancer and recombinant erythropoietin is widely used to treat anaemia in patients undergoing chemotherapy and improves quality of life. However, data from a recent Cochrane meta-analysis indicate that, currently, there is insufficient evidence to recommend the use of erythropoietin in the pre- and perioperative period in colorectal cancer surgery [33].

There are also concerns pertaining to administration of erythropoietin-stimulating agents (ESAs) to patients with cancer. These have been associated with increased risk of veno-thromboembolism and mortality by some. In the USA, the Federal Drug Agency (FDA) issued a recommendation in 2008 substantially limiting the use of ESAs to treat anaemia in cancer patients, indicating that they be restricted to advanced cancer patients. National Institute for Health and Clinical Excellence (NICE) has also indicated that ESAs should only be used in patients with an Hb less than 8 g/dL or where blood transfusions are inappropriate. We would therefore regard it as inappropriate to use ESAs in patients with iron deficiency anaemia who are to undergo elective colorectal cancer surgery. Further multi-centre randomised trials are needed to define how best to treat anaemia avoiding transfusion prior to major colorectal surgery.

Nutrition

Poor nutritional status is associated with poorer outcome after major surgery. Hiram Studley first reported this in the 1930s where preoperative weight loss and higher postoperative complications were linked [37]. A proportion of colorectal cancer patients would be nutritionally challenged at the time of presentation. It is established that both infectious and non-infectious complications and even mortality are significantly increased in the malnourished patient [38].

Table 2.4 Nutritional Risk Score (NRS)

		Mild	Moderate	Severe
		1	2	3
Age (years)		>70		
Nutritional status	BMI		18.5–20.5	<18.5
	Food intake [%]	50–75	25–50	<25
	Weight loss <5%	3 months	2 months	1 month
Disease severity	Example	Hip fracture	Major surgery	BM Transplant

Table 2.5 Nutritional Risk Score and postoperative morbidity

	NRS	Complications (%)	Infections (%)
Minor surgery	<3	6	2
	>3	10	7
Major surgery	<3	23	13
	>3	58	35

An assessment of a patient's nutritional status is not straightforward and currently there is a lack of standardisation in the definition of nutritional depletion and there is no consensus on the best method for assessing the nutritional status of hospitalised patients. Multiple factors have been found to be associated with poor nutritional status and it is perhaps not one particular system that matters over another but that some assessment and consideration for intervention is given when nutritional depletion is thought to be present.

A recent retrospective single-centre study from Italy assessed 1,410 major gastrointestinal cancer operations and found advanced age, weight loss, low serum albumin and a lack of nutritional support (and pancreatic surgery) to be independent risk factors for postoperative complications. Others have identified pre-albumin, transthyretin, BMI, oral intake, disease severity, bio-impedance, hand-grip strength and anthropometry measurements (e.g., triceps skin-fold) as risk factors. Multiple systems exist to predict nutritional 'risk' including subjective global assessment (SGA); mini-nutritional assessment; Nutrition Risk Index and Nutrition Risk Score (NRS) [39].

Recently, the Nutrition Risk Score (see Tables 2.4 and 2.5) has shown some promise in the identification of at-risk individuals. This score is based upon age, disease severity and nutritional status (BMI, food intake, weight loss >5% time) and where three or more factors are positive then this is associated with poorer outcome in a major surgery [40].

Where patients are identified as nutritionally 'at-risk', then the most suitable preoperative intervention is the initiation of oral nutritional supplements and a dietician should be involved in the decision-making process. Preoperative oral nutritional supplements should be given to patients with insufficient food intake and given preferably before admission to hospital [41]. The benefits of oral nutritional supplements and enteral tube feeding have been confirmed in meta-analysis [42]. The evidence for how long oral nutritional supplements should be given pre- and postoperatively is less clear but is suggested to be 5–7 days before surgery and for 5–7 days after uncomplicated surgery [41]. The most appropriate supplement is a standard whole protein formula for most patients but more recently, the role of 'immunonutrition' with formulas containing arginine, omega-3 fatty acids and ribonucleic acid (RNA) has been assessed and evidence is building for its role in major abdominal cancer surgery and after severe trauma [41]. It is imperative that the data be interpreted in the context of individual patient's risk since specialty formulas appear most beneficial in patients at risk of subsequent complications or those with significant pre-existing malnutrition. Preoperative immunonutrition in malnourished patients has been more beneficial than perioperative conventional nutritional support.

Where severe nutritional risk is identified (e.g., weight loss >10–15%/6 months; BMI <18.5; Subjective Global Assessment Grade C; serum albumin <30 [with normal renal/hepatic function]) surgery should be delayed where possible and nutritional deficits corrected as soon as this risk is identified. This group is unlikely to follow a complete enhanced recovery after surgery (ERAS) pathway although some components would still be suitable. The role of other nutritional supports including parenteral feeding and enteral tube feeding is beyond the scope of this chapter.

Obesity

Obesity is a significant problem among most of the European patient population and with this comes obesity-related disease. Obese patients have significantly more surgical site infections and soft tissue complications after surgery and have a greater proportion of deep venous thromboses, incidence of postoperative lung dysfunction and metabolic disturbance postoperatively. In some cases, elective surgery can be postponed to allow weight loss by medical means or bariatric surgery; however, in the colorectal cancer population this is not feasible.

Hypertension

Hypertension treatment is associated with a reduced mortality from stroke and coronary heart disease. In surgical patients, however, it is apparent in the literature that if a patient has a systolic blood pressure below 180 mmHg and a diastolic blood pressure less than 110 mmHg (stage 1 or stage 2) then high blood pressure is not an independent risk factor for cardiovascular complications in the perioperative period [10]. Despite this finding, identification of hypertension in the pre-assessment clinic is an opportunity to initiate treatment via the patient's general practitioner even though it is unlikely to have an effect upon the overall outcome of the planned surgery.

Where a systolic and diastolic blood pressure is identified as over 180 and 110 mmHg, respectively (stage 3 hypertension), then postponing surgery to initiate or optimise anti-hypertensive medications may be merited if the risk of delaying surgery is acceptable. Nevertheless, one randomized trial was unable to demonstrate a benefit to delaying surgery for a diastolic blood pressure between 110 and 130 mmHg in a group with no previous MI, unstable or severe angina pectoris, renal failure, pregnancy-induced hypertension, left ventricular hypertrophy, previous coronary revascularization, aortic stenosis, preoperative dysrhythmias, conduction defects or stroke [10, 43]. The trial patients received 10 mg of nifedipine delivered intranasally to rapidly control blood pressure and the control group had surgery postponed and had in-patient blood pressure control and no significant differences in postoperative morbidity was observed. This suggests that Stage 3 hypertension on the day of surgery in the absence of significant cardiovascular morbidity need not delay surgery.

Patients taking angiotensin-converting enzyme (ACE) inhibitors and angiotensin II (ATII) receptor antagonists are at higher risk of intraoperative hypotension and reports vary on the effect upon cardiac and renal complications in the perioperative period and this has prompted a move for ACE I and ATII receptor inhibitors to be withheld on the morning of surgery [10] with the recommendation that once a patient is deemed euvolaemic postoperatively that they be restarted owing to concerns regarding perioperative renal dysfunction.

Diabetes

It is well established that poor glucose control in the perioperative period is an independent predictor of postoperative infection and mortality independent of diabetic status [44] countering the historical acceptance of relatively high glucose levels in the perioperative period. The control of blood glucose concentration is therefore more crucial than making a diagnosis of diabetes.

Nevertheless, while clinical trials demonstrate the harmful effects of perioperative hyperglycaemia, the ideal target for cardiovascular benefit of intraoperative and postoperative glycaemic control are not yet entirely clear. In addition, tight glycaemic control may exert a cost in terms of increased incidence of severe hypoglycaemia. The ultimate goal in the management of diabetic patients is to achieve equivalent outcomes as those patients without diabetes.

Diabetes mellitus is common in the colorectal surgery population and its presence should heighten suspicion of occult coronary artery disease (CAD) as both CAD and myocardial ischaemia and heart failure are more likely in patients with diabetes mellitus. The requirement for insulin in diabetes is an independent cardiac risk factor in the Lee index. Mortality rates in diabetic patients are estimated to be up to five times greater than in non-diabetic patients. This has been attributed to end-organ damage caused by the disease. Chronic complications resulting in microangiopathy (retinopathy, nephropathy and neuropathy) and macroangiopathy (atherosclerosis) directly increase the need for surgical intervention and the occurrence of surgical complications due to infections and vasculopathies. In general, infections account for 66% of postoperative complications and nearly one quarter of perioperative deaths in patients with diabetes. Data suggest that impaired leukocyte function, including altered chemotaxis and phagocytic activity, may underlie this finding.

Optimisation of glucose control preoperatively is the ideal and should be done in cooperation with the patient's general practitioner and endocrinologist/diabetic liaison nurse and individualised to the patient. Comprehensive preoperative assessment and intensive intraoperative and postoperative management by a multidisciplinary team are recommended. It is estimated that one quarter of diabetic patients are unaware that they have the disease hence it is prudent to screen all patients undergoing major colorectal surgery by checking glycosylated haemoglobin (HbA1c or A1C). A recent novel study in colorectal cancer patients showed that every fourth patient undergoing colorectal surgery without known diabetes had an elevated HbA1c as an indicator of glucose intolerance. These patients also had a higher glucose level after surgery, higher CRP levels and more complications, in particular infectious complications. [45]

In addition to standard preoperative information, details of a patient's current diabetes management should be documented, e.g., duration of treatment, specific medication regimen and issues with insulin resistance or hypersensitivity. Preoperative measurement of HbA1c may identify patients at higher risk of poor glycaemic control and postoperative complications and general practitioners may be able to offer this information during the preoperative work-up.

In general, on the day of surgery, patients on oral hypoglycaemic agents are advised to discontinue them owing to their potential to cause hypoglycaemia. In addition, sulfonylureas have been associated with interfering with ischemic myocardial pre-conditioning and may theoretically increase the risk of perioperative myocardial ischaemia and infarction. Metformin should be discontinued preoperatively because of the risk of developing lactic acidosis. For such patients, short-acting insulin may be administered subcutaneously as a sliding scale or as a continuous infusion, to maintain optimal glucose control, depending on the type and duration of surgery. Patients will be advised of these modifications at the pre-assessment clinic. Maintenance insulin may be continued, based on the history of glucose concentrations and the discretion of the endocrinologist/diabetic liaison team.

Smoking and Alcohol Intake

Smoking and high alcohol intakes are important risk factors for perioperative morbidity in all elective and emergency surgery. The most common perioperative complications related to smoking are impaired wound healing, wound infection and cardiopulmonary complications. Even in young smokers, reduced pulmonary capacity, increased mucus production and reduced ciliary function are recorded [46].

All patients presenting for surgery should be questioned regarding smoking and hazardous drinking as clear benefit is obtained by intensive interventions to encourage their cessation as this translates to benefit by significantly reducing the incidence of several serious postoperative complications, including wound and cardiopulmonary complications and infections. The duration of these interventions can, however, be between 3 and 8 weeks or longer meaning that patients requiring prompt surgery may not gain this advantage [47].

Patient Education and Conditioning of Expectations

The colorectal surgery patient is faced with high psychological and physical stress levels and the threat of significant disruption in a number of valued role areas: work function and career, as a parent and spouse, community involvement, recreational activities, gender identity, possible stoma and no longer being a 'well person'. This may lead to depression and lowered self-esteem as well as placing additional strain on the social support systems that are already trying to cope with the surgery process itself. This can be reduced with patient education and conditioning of expectations.

Particularly in cancer patients, it would be regarded as more appropriate for information to be given about perioperative care in enhanced recovery in a subsequent separate session from the appointment when the diagnosis is discussed, as a distressed patient is less likely to respond to attempts to educate and modify expectations.

The enhanced recovery consensus is that preoperative information is beneficial and patient education should describe the patient's journey and condition expectations for the period of hospitalisation. Intensive preoperative patient information facilitates postoperative recovery, reduces anxiety and pain, and improves postoperative self-care and symptom management, particularly in patients who exhibit the most denial and the highest levels of anxiety [48–52]. Several meta-analyses have demonstrated the benefits of preoperative education outcome [53, 54].

Delivering information during pre-assessment appears to be more effective than in the immediate preoperative period [55, 56] Patient education includes emphasising the importance of a patient's role in his or her own recovery and a clear explanation of what is to happen encourages adherence to the ERAS care pathway as compliance is currently believed to be central to a successful programme [57]. Patients should be engaged in their recovery by being given tasks to perform and targets to meet during the postoperative period, for instance food intake and mobilisation, and criteria that should be met to permit discharge from hospital. Suitable discharge criteria comprise the ability to tolerate solid food, to be able to fully mobilise, oral analgesia adequately resolving the pain and flatus and/or faeces are passed indicating gut function is maintained, the patient is afebrile and agrees for discharge [2]. If criteria for discharge are not adequately explained this can result in a delayed discharge [58]. Social aspects of a patient's care may hinder the patient's timely discharge. Often patients are medically fit for discharge but have insufficient social circumstances to support their discharge or they may be unwilling to be discharged despite suitable medical fitness [57]. Pre-assessment should aim to determine what social aspects are deficient that may delay discharge. Wherever possible, these factors should be modified preoperatively in cooperation with social workers, general practitioners and occupational therapists.

As yet there is no single definitive method of information giving that will suit all patients or enhanced recovery teams to achieve preoperative optimisation, but basic guidelines for patients are useful and should be both oral and written (and easily readable) forms for the intended audience [59]. The use of patient diaries may benefit patient understanding, motivation and assist in audit of patient compliance. There may also be benefit in showing patients and relatives the ward onto which they will be admitted and familiarising them with its layout as part of the pre-admission process. Patients are likely to recover more quickly in an elective-only environment and the ward should be designed to facilitate the feeling of security, encourage independence and allow free access to food preparation and self-care facilities [60].

Setting realistic goals and discussing potential morbidity is also important and has a positive impact upon recovery [61]. 'Informative preparations' can be both 'procedural' and 'sensory information' indicating what the patient will see, hear, feel and taste. Hendry reported that about half of unselected patients were able to have their intravenous fluids removed the day following surgery and about half were able to get out of bed on the day of surgery and about two-thirds were able to resume a full diet on the day after surgery [62]. Morbidity is reduced overall and readmission rates around 10% and reoperation rates below 8% are quoted in recent studies [63, 64]. Post-discharge expectations should be clarified; King reported 58% of patients undergoing open colorectal surgery felt fully recovered at 12 months compared to almost 90% of laparoscopic surgery patients within an enhanced recovery programme [64].

Despite preoperative education being clearly beneficial, how well a patient processes this information depends upon their information comprehension, recall ability (attention span, memory capacity, age, past experiences, educational level and coping style) and attitude [65]. Standardising an educational program for patients that is provided by nurses may therefore not always address an individual patient's needs. Nonetheless, experienced pre-assessment nursing staff will be able to respond to this and will not assume patient information needs, tailoring education according to an individual's knowledge and needs, whilst still emphasising the crucial aspects of ERAS that a patient participates in.

Evidence is evolving for how the host response to surgery may be modified by patient psychology and psychological interventions exerting influences upon immune function, wound healing and short-term postoperative recovery [66]. Of interest a link between molecular markers [vascular endothelial growth factor (VEGF) pre- and postoperatively] in colorectal cancer and anxiety/depression and functional well-being levels has been identified and psychological intervention in a randomised clinical trial in advanced breast cancer patients, natural killer (NK) cell function was elevated [67, 68].

Preparing patients for surgery by education and conditioning of expectations may therefore induce physical changes that will improve outcome. Factors that are considered relevant are: the patient's attitude towards surgery and enhanced recovery and pre-morbid personality significantly influence emotional status during the decision-making process. In turn, emotions have a direct effect on 'stress' hormones and these modulate immune function: Personality type has been found to influence hospital stay and it is likely to exert an effect upon pain threshold. In a recent study postoperative morbidity and extroversion were predictors of length of stay [69, 70]. Postoperative anxiety and depression are closely linked to preoperative levels using validated psychological questionnaires and are related to postoperative quality of life [69]. Preoperative health behaviour can also influence outcome, including immune and endocrine function, wound healing and overall postoperative rehabilitation. When patients are under stress, they may increase negative short-term destructive coping behaviours including smoking, alcohol and caloric intake and these can have a deleterious effect on not only immune and neuroendocrine function, but also on postoperative physical recovery.

Cognitive behavioural techniques, hypnosis, relaxation techniques, visualisation, imagery and psychosocial interventions have been employed in preoperative patients with significant benefit to outcomes however; these techniques are beyond the scope of this chapter.

Summary

- Preoperative assessment is essential to determine and modify patient co-morbidity prior to surgery to improve recovery and reduce complications.
- Cardiopulmonary function can be optimised in high-risk patients in close liaison with a cardiologist and an anaesthetist.
- Attention to a patient's functional capacity and cardiac risk factors can identify patients requiring further specialist assessment prior to surgery.
- Poor nutrition should be addressed preoperatively, where possible, and oral nutritional supplement will be suitable for most patients.
- Anaemia should be treated preoperatively, where possible, to reduce the need for perioperative blood transfusion.
- Conditioning patient expectations prior to the operation improves patient recovery and reduces anxiety.

Conclusions

Enhanced recovery aims to reduce the surgical stress response, improve the quality of recovery and reduce complications. Pre-assessment is first step in this process. Providing appropriate information to patients ensures co-operation and reduces anxiety. Pre-assessment ensures modifiable risks can be adjusted and appropriate investigation performed to permit optimisation of a patient's condition for surgery. An optimised and informed patient can expect a more rapid and better quality recovery.

References

1. Wind J, Polle SW, Fung Kon Jin PHP, et al. Systematic review of enhanced recovery programmes in colonic surgery. Br J Surg. 2006;93(7):800–9.
2. Varadhan KK, Neal KR, Dejong CHC, et al. The enhanced recovery after surgery (ERAS) pathway for patients undergoing major elective open colorectal surgery: a meta-analysis of randomized controlled trials. Clin Nutr. 2010. doi:10.1016/j.clnu.2010.01.004.

3. Gouvas N, Tan E, Windsor A, Xynos E, Tekkis PP. Fast-track vs. standard care in colorectal surgery: a meta-analysis update. Int J Colorectal Dis. 2009;24:1119–31.
4. Lassen K, Soop M, Nygren J, et al. Consensus review of optimal perioperative care in colorectal surgery. Arch Surg. 2009;144(10):961–9.
5. Department of Health. Cancer waiting targets – a guide (Version 5). Department of Health. From http://www.performance.doh.gov.uk/cancerwaits (2006). Retrieved 6 May 2009.
6. Halaszynski TM, Juda R, Silverman DG. Optimizing postoperative outcomes with efficient preoperative assessment and management. Crit Care Med. 2004;32(4):S76–86.
7. Kheterpal S, O'Reilly M, Englesbe MJ, et al. Preoperative and intraoperative predictors of cardiac adverse events after general, vascular, and urological surgery. Anesthesiology. 2009;110:58–66.
8. National Confidential Enquiry Into Patient Outcome And Death. Accessed Mar 2010 www.ncepod.org.uk
9. Kehlet H. Multimodal approach to postoperative recovery. Curr Opin Crit Care. 2009; 15:355–8.
10. Focused Update on Perioperative Beta Blockade Incorporated Into the ACC/AHA. Guidelines on perioperative cardiovascular evaluation and care for noncardiac surgery: a report of the American College of Cardiology Foundation/American Heart Association Task Force on Practice Guidelines. Circulation. 2009;120:e169–276.
11. Poldermans D, Bax JJ, Boersma E, et al. Guidelines for pre-operative cardiac risk assessment and perioperative cardiac management in non-cardiac surgery: the Task Force for Preoperative Cardiac Risk Assessment and Perioperative Cardiac Management in Non-cardiac Surgery of the European Society of Cardiology (ESC) and endorsed by the European Society of Anaesthesiology (ESA). Eur J Anaesthesiol. 2010;27(2):92–137.
12. Poldermans D, Bax JJ, Boersma E, et al. Guidelines for pre-operative cardiac risk assessment and perioperative cardiac management in non-cardiac surgery. Eur Heart J. 2009; 30(22):2769–812.
13. Lee TH, Marcantonio ER, Mangione CM, et al. Derivation and prospective validation of a simple index for prediction of cardiac risk of major noncardiac surgery. Circulation. 1999;100(10):1043–9.
14. Boersma E, Kertai MD, Schouten O, et al. Perioperative cardiovascular mortality in noncardiac surgery: validation of the Lee cardiac risk index. Am J Med. 2005;118(10):1134–41.
15. Hlatky MA, Boineau RE, Higginbotham MB, et al. A brief self-administered questionnaire to determine functional capacity (the Duke Activity Status Index). Am J Cardiol. 1989;64(10):651–4.
16. Fletcher GF, Balady GJ, Amsterdam EA, et al. Exercise standards for testing and training: a statement for healthcare professionals from the American Heart Association. Circulation. 2001;104(14):1694–740.
17. Biccard BM. Relationship between the inability to climb two flights of stairs and outcome after major non-cardiac surgery: implications for the preoperative assessment of functional capacity. Anaesthesia. 2005;60/6:588–93.
18. Wiklund RA, Stein HD, Rosenbaum SH. Activities of daily living and cardiovascular complications following elective, noncardiac surgery. Yale J Biol Med. 2001;74:75–87.
19. Amsworth BE et al. Compendium of physical activities: an update of activity indices. Med Sci Sports Med. 2000;32(9 S):S498–504.
20. Byrne NM, Hills AP, Hunter GR, et al. Metabolic equivalent; one size does not fit all. J Appl Physiol. 2005;99:1112–9.
21. Davies SJ, Wilson RJT. Preoperative optimization of the high-risk surgical patient. Br J Anaesth. 2004;93:121–8.
22. Older P, Smith R, Courtney P, Hone R. Preoperative optimization of the high-risk surgical patient of cardiac failure and ischemia in elderly patients by cardiopulmonary exercise testing. Chest. 1993;104:701–4.
23. Lawrence VA, Cornell JE, Smetana GW. Clinical guidelines. Strategies to reduce postoperative pulmonary complications after noncardiothoracic surgery: systematic review for the American College of Physicians. Ann Intern Med. 2006;144(8):596–608.

24. Goodnough LT, Shander A, Spivak JL, et al. Detection, evaluation, and management of anemia in the elective surgical patient. Anesth Analg. 2005;101(6):1858–61.
25. Dunne JR, Gannon CJ, Osbin TM, et al. Preoperative anaemia in colon cancer: assessment of risk factors. Am Surg. 2002;68(6):582–7.
26. Kim J, Konyalim V, Hughn R, et al. Identification of predictive factors for perioperative blood transfusion in colorectal resection patients. Int J Colorectal Dis. 2007;22:1493–7.
27. Amato A, Pescatori M. Perioperative blood transfusion for the recurrence of colorectal cancer. Cochrane Database Syst Rev. 2006;1:art no: CD005033.
28. Busch DR, Hop NC, Marquet RL, et al. The effect of blood transfusion on survival after surgery for colorectal cancer. Eur J Cancer. 1995;31A(7–8):1226–8.
29. Kranenburg WM, Hermans J, Van de Velde CJH, et al. For Cancer Recurrence and Blood Transfusion Group: Perioperative blood transfusion with or without allogenic leukocytes relate to survival and not to cancer recurrence. Br J Surg. 2001;88:267–72.
30. American Society of Anaesthesiologists: Standards, Guidelines and statements: Accessed Mar 2010. www.asahq.org/publicationsAndServices/sgstoc.htm.
31. Lidder PG, Sanders G, Whitehead E, et al. Preoperative oral iron supplementation reduces blood transfusion in colorectal surgery – a prospective, randomised, controlled trial. Ann R Coll Surg Engl. 2007;89:418.
32. Edwards TG, Noble EJ, Durran A, et al. Randomised clinical trial of preoperative intravenous iron sucrose to reduce blood transfusion in anaemic patients after colorectal cancer surgery. BJS. 2009;96(10):1122–8.
33. Devon KM, McLeod RS. Pre and perioperative erythropoeitin for reducing allogeneic blood transfusions in colorectal cancer surgery. Cochrane Database Syst Rev. 2009(1). doi:10.1002/14651858.CD007148.pub2. Art. No.: CD007148.
34. Okuyama A et al. Preoperative iron supplementation and intraoperative transfusion during colorectal cancer surgery. Surg Today. 2005;35(1):35–40.
35. Beris P, Munoz M, Garcia-Erce JA, et al. Perioperative anaemia management: consensus statement on the role of intravenous iron. Br J Anaesth. 2008;100(5):599–604.
36. Bhandal N, Russell R. Intravenous versus oral iron therapy for post-partum patients. BJOG. 2006;113(11):1248–52.
37. Studley H. Percentage of weight loss: a basic indication of surgical risk in patients with chronic peptic ulcer. JAMA. 1936;106(6):458–60.
38. Correia MITD, Wartzberg DC. The impact of malnutrition on morbidity, mortality, length of hospital stay and costs evaluated through a multivariate model analysis. Clin Nutr. 2003;22(3):235–9.
39. Bozzetti F, Gianotti L, Braga M, Di Carlo V, Mariani L. Post-operative complications in gastrointestinal cancer patients: the joint role of the nutritional status and the nutritional support. Clin Nutr. 2007;26(6):698–709.
40. Kondrup J, Rasmussen HO, Hamberg O, et al. Nutritional Risk Screening [NRS 2002]: a new method based on an analysis of controlled clinical trials. Clin Nutr. 2003;22(3):321–36.
41. Weimann A, Braga M, Harsanyi L, et al. ESPEN Guidelines on enteral nutrition: surgery including organ transplantation. Clin Nutr. 2006;25(2):224–44.
42. Stratton RJ, Elia M. Who benefits from nutritional support: what is the evidence? Eur J Gastroenterol Hepatol. 2007;19(5):353–8.
43. Weksler N, Klein M, Szendro G, et al. The dilemma of immediate preoperative hypertension: to treat and operate, or to postpone surgery? J Clin Anesth. 2003;15(3):179–83.
44. Doenst T, Wijesundera D, Karkouti K, et al. Hyperglycaemia during cardiopulmonary bypass is an independent risk factor for mortality in patients undergoing cardiac surgery. J Thorac Cardiovasc Surg. 2005;130:1144.
45. Gustafsson UO et al. Haemoglobin A1c as a predictor of postoperative hyperglycaemia and complications after major colorectal surgery. Br J Surg. 2009;96(11):1358–64.
46. Hans P, Marechal J, Maheu B, et al. Effect of propofol and sevoflurane on coughing in smokers and non-smokers awakening from general anaesthesia at the end of a cervical spine surgery. Br J Anaesth. 2008;101:731–7.
47. Tønnesen H, Neilson PR, Lauritzen JB, Møller AM. Smoking and alcohol intervention before surgery: evidence for best practice. Br J Anaesth. 2009;102(3):297–306.

48. Maessen JMC, Dejong CHC, Kessels AGH, von Meyenfeldt MF. Length of stay: an inappropriate readout of the success of enhanced recovery programs. World J Surg. 2008;32: 971–5.
49. Kiecolt-Glaser JK, Page GG, Marrucha PT, MacCallum RC, Glaser R. Psychological influences on surgical recovery perspectives from pscychthoreumoimmunology. Am Psycho. 1996;53(11):1209–18.
50. Egbert LD, Bartt G, Welch C, Bartlett M. Reduction of postoperative pain by encouragement and instruction of patients: a study of doctor-patient rapport. N Engl J Med. 1964;270:825–7.
51. TM Halasz ynski, Juda R, Silverman DG. Optimizing postoperative outcomes with efficient preoperative assessment and management. Crit Care Med. 2004;32(4 Suppl):S76–86.
52. Forster AJ, Clark HD, Menard A, Dupuis N, Chernish R, Chandok N, et al. Effect of a nurse team coordinator on outcomes for hospitalized medicine patients. Am J Med. 2005;118(10):1148–53.
53. Disbrow EA, Bernett HL, Owings JT. Effect of preoperative suggestion on postoperative gastrointestinal motility. West J Med. 1993;153(5):438–92.
54. Blay N, Donoghue J. The effect of pre-admission education on domiciliary recovery following laparoscopic cholecystectomy. Aust J Adv Nurs. 2005;22(4):14–9.
55. Devine EC. Effects of psychoeducation care for adult surgical patients: a meta-analysis of 191 studies. Patient Educ Couns. 1992;19:129–42.
56. Shuldman C. A review of the impact of preoperative education on recovery from surgery. Int J Nurs Stud. 1999;36:171–7.
57. Maessen J, Dejong CHC, Hausel J, et al. A protocol is not enough to implement an enhanced recovery programme for colorectal resection. Br J Surg. 2007;94:224–31.
58. Delaney CP, Zutshi M, Senagore AJ, et al. Prospective, randomized, controlled trial between a pathway of controlled rehabilitation with early ambulation and diet and traditional postoperative care and laparotomy and intestinal resection. Dis Colon Rectum. 2003;46:851–9.
59. Billyard J, Boyne S, Watson J. Implementing an enhanced recovery programme in a district general hospital. Gastrointest Nurs. 2007;5(9):32–9.
60. Williams AM, Irurita VF. Enhancing the therapeutic potential of hospital environments by increasing the personal control and emotional comfort of hospitalized patients. Appl Nurs Res. 2005;18(1):22–8.
61. Prokop CK, Bradley LA, Burish TG, Anderson KO, Fox JE. Psychological preparation for stressful medical and dental procedures. In: Prokop CK, Bradley LA, editors. Health psychology: clinical methods and research. New York: Macmillan; 1991. p. 159–96.
62. Hendry PO, Hausel J, Nygren J, et al. Determinants of outcome after colorectal resection within an enhanced recovery programme. Br J Surg. 2009;96:197–205.
63. Andersen J, Hjort-Jakobsen D, Christiansen PS, Kehlet H. Readmission rates after a planned hospital stay of 2 versus 3 days in fast-track colonic surgery. Br J Surg. 2007;94:890–3.
64. King PM, Blazeby JM, Ewings P, Kennedy RH. Detailed evaluation of functional recovery following laparoscopic or open surgery for colorectal cancer within an enhanced recovery programme. Int J Colorectal Dis. 2008;23:795–800.
65. Oetker-Black SL, Taunton RL. Evaluation of a self-efficacy scale for preoperative patients. AORN J. 1994;60:43–50.
66. Kiecolt-Glaser JK, Page GG, Marucha PT, MacCallum RC, Glaser R. Psychological influences on surgical recovery: Perspectives from psychoneuroimmunology. Am Psychol. 1998;53:1209–18.
67. Sharma A, Greenman J, Sharp DM, Walker LG, Monson JR. Vascular endothelial growth factor and psychosocial factors in colorectal cancer. Psychooncology. 2008;17(1):66–73.
68. Eremin O, Walker MB, Simpson E, et al. Immuno-modulatory effects of relaxation training and guided imagery in women with locally advanced breast cancer undergoing multimodality therapy: a randomised controlled trial. Breast. 2009;18(1):17–25.
69. Sharma A, Sharp DM, Walker LG, Monson JR. Predictors of early postoperative quality of life after elective resection for colorectal cancer. Ann Surg Oncol. 2007;14(12):3435–42.
70. Sharma A, Sharp DM, Walker LG, Monson JR. Patient personality predicts postoperative stay after colorectal cancer resection. Colorectal Dis. 2008;10(2):151–6.

Chapter 3
The Metabolic Stress Response and Enhanced Recovery

Olle Ljungqvist

The Metabolic Response to Injury

Injury and surgery immediately cause a series of stress responses in the body. The most important reactions involve the release of stress hormones and cytokines. The level of these reactions is related to the amount of stress inflicted. With greater stress, increasingly stronger reactions cause more marked catabolic reactions. Central to all these reactions is the loss of the normal anabolic actions of insulin, i.e., the development of insulin resistance [1]. Excessive catabolic reactions are generally not beneficial for the body and a state of catabolism continuously breaks down muscle tissue and prolongs recovery. Hence a key aspect of enhancing recovery after surgery is related to minimising the negative metabolic effects by reducing the catabolic responses and having the patient return to a balanced metabolism again.

Insulin is the most important anabolic hormone in the body. Insulin regulates glucose metabolism keeping it within very tight limits in healthy people. Insulin ensures that glucose levels are normalised shortly after food intake by activating rapid glucose uptake in muscle and fat along with glucose loading in the liver as glycogen. Other organs and cells have a transient increase of glucose uptake since they take up glucose in relation to the prevailing glucose level. Insulin also controls protein metabolism primarily by reducing protein breakdown in the muscle, but also by supporting protein synthesis in the presence of amino acids. In insulin-sensitive cells, primarily muscle and fat, insulin acts via specific receptors on the cell surface of these cells. Inside these insulin-sensitive cells specific signalling pathways are activated for facilitating the anabolic reactions such as glycogen storage and protein synthesis in muscle or the blocking of lipolysis in fat cells.

O. Ljungqvist
Department of Surgery, Örebro University Hospital, Örebro, Sweden

N. Francis et al. (eds.), *Manual of Fast Track Recovery for Colorectal Surgery*,
Enhanced Recovery, DOI 10.1007/978-0-85729-953-6_3,
© Springer-Verlag London Limited 2012

With any major injury to the body, these actions by insulin are overrun by the release of the stress hormones and the inflammatory reactions mediated by cytokines. Amino acids, free fatty acids and glucose is released to the blood stream as a reaction to injury. Substrate metabolism also changes and the body starts to consume fat over glucose. In medium- to large-size operations such as colorectal surgery these reactions are reversible and studies have shown that if the insulin is infused in sufficient amounts to bring down glucose to normal levels, the rest of metabolism is also normalised [2]. Hence protein breakdown is normalised, and free fatty acid levels and substrate oxidation return to normal once the effects of insulin on metabolism are reinstituted. From a clinical point of view it seems that infusion of sufficient insulin to normalise glucose levels can be used as an end point target to achieve these reactions.

Insulin Resistance and Complications After Surgery

In recent years it has become evident that the changes in metabolism and the excessive catabolism is a main cause for many of the common complications occurring after surgery. Hyperglycaemia is one such cause of complications and the development in surgical hyperglycaemia is similar to that described for hyperglycaemia in diabetic patients [3] Hence some of key characteristics of hyperglycaemia are an increase in glucose production, a relative reduction in glucose uptake in the periphery and the loss of activation of glucose transporters and glycogen storage in response to insulin stimulation. These changes also occur in type 2 diabetes. With insulin resistance and the development of hyperglycaemia, the main mechanism for glucose uptake into the large depots in muscle and fat is shut off. Instead glucose uptake is markedly increased in the organs and cells that take up glucose in relation to the prevailing glucose level. These cells include blood cells, renal cells, endothelial cells and neural cells. Whilst glucose uptake is largely enhanced, these cells have no way of blocking glucose uptake in response to this rapidly developing stress. In addition, these cells have no storage capacity for glucose. This leaves only glycolysis as the sole metabolic pathway remaining open for glucose. This eventually causes problems for these cells. With massive glucose inflow to the mitochondria eventually the oxidative capacity is overrun and oxygen free radicals are produced. This eventually may cause changes in the cell metabolism that renders changes in gene expression and signalling. These reactions occur in many cells such as endothelial tissue, kidney, nerve cells and blood cells. These are also the key cells involved in many of the most common complications such as cardiovascular complications, renal failure, neuropathy and infections. Muscle is also affected by surgical stress and fatigue is a very common postoperative problem. This fatigue can be explained by a combination of disturbed intracellular glucose metabolism and protein catabolic reaction causing muscle breakdown. Recent studies have shown that the main pathways for insulin signalling are disturbed after surgical stress and this blocks the normal actions of insulin in muscle cells [4, 5]. This is also true for the fat cells in which pathways of insulin are disturbed while pathways enhancing inflammation are up regulated [6]. The heart is another muscle that is vulnerable to stress and metabolic disturbances and insulin-resistant states. Insulin has also been shown to be a key hormone for tissue healing and hence a state of insulin resistance is accompanied by worse healing capacity [7].

Many of the complications in surgical stress are similar to those occurring in patients with diabetes. Interestingly, the changes occurring in postoperative glucose metabolism are also very similar to those found in diabetes. Whilst in diabetes the changes in glucose metabolism and the accompanying complications usually develop slowly over the years, the change in stress-induced glucose metabolism is rapidly established within minutes, and the complications occur within the first week of surgery.

Studies of postoperative patients with moderate stress (APACHE II around 10–15) have shown that controlling glucose levels with insulin impacts outcome by reducing the development of some of the more common complications in the surgical ICU [8, 9] In addition, observational studies in patients undergoing colorectal surgery and treated in surgical wards with a lower glucose level had fewer complications than those with only slightly higher levels [10].

Whilst in recent years the focus in postoperative metabolism has been on glucose, there is an abundant literature from earlier years showing that negative protein balance is also detrimental to recovery after surgery. Protein balance is also under strong influence of insulin. Hence, in insulin-resistant states, protein balance becomes negative and in particular protein breakdown occurs in muscle. The main effect of insulin is reducing protein breakdown in muscle, while protein synthesis is mainly stimulated by the presence of amino acids [11]. In stress-induced insulin resistance, treatment with insulin can counteract protein losses [2, 12] and support tissue healing [13]. Smaller experimental studies in humans clearly suggest that retaining insulin action is a key to anabolism and is likely to play a role in the avoiding complications after surgery. In larger clinical studies this notion has been supported in a large randomised trial of patients after mainly thoracic surgery. These patients were given a combination of enteral and parenteral nutrition and when given insulin to normalise glucose to 4.5–6.0 mmol/L, the authors reported a marked reduction in complications that affected cells sensitive to hyperglycaemia and a marked reduction in mortality. In a follow-up large multi-centre trial of patients under greater stress, a similar treatment had a small but opposite effect with a slightly higher mortality. These seemingly conflicting findings may potentially be explained by some main differences between the trials. The first one studied patients under less stress than the second study. This is obvious from the about three times higher mortality rate in the second trial. In situations of increasingly greater stress, the effect of insulin eventually vanishes and may even be counter-effective [9]. Secondly, the extent to which the protocol was followed differed between the two trials. In the first one performed in a single unit, the protocol compliance was very good and the variation in glucose levels was substantially less than in the second trial.

Some Special Risk Groups

The malnourished patient is at particular risk of complications, and will risk having a slower recovery [14]. It is therefore important to identify patients who are malnourished or at risk of becoming malnourished and it is advised to inform the patient the importance of eating normal food and also to be liberal with providing nutritional supplements during the period before the operation [15].

The patient with diabetes is another patient with higher risks of complications. These patients are at risk of being catabolic from the very start if their diabetes is not under control. In addition, diabetic patients become even more insulin resistant after surgery. While some reports indicate that it may be the peak glucose value that is related to major outcomes after surgery, it is also clear that diabetic patients more often reach higher glucose levels after surgery compared with non diabetics [16]. Patients with cancer coming for surgery also have a higher prevalence of disturbed glucose metabolism, even if they have not been diagnosed with diabetes. This is indicated by a novel study in colorectal surgical patients, showing that every fourth patient coming in for colorectal surgery without knowledge of diabetes had an elevated HbA1c as an indicator of glucose intolerance [10]. These patients also had a higher glucose level after surgery, higher CRP levels and more complications, in particular infectious complications. This is not all that surprising since cancer is known to cause insulin resistance.

The surgeon usually meets the patient a few weeks before the patient is about to be operated. Many of the patients will have cancer surgery, and some will have radiation or chemotherapy, but most of them will be planned for surgery as quickly as possible. In most units the operation can be done within a few weeks. This allows the patient to prepare metabolically and for the surgeon to institute appropriate treatments.

Preoperative Nutritional Support

In the 2–3 weeks before the operation, the patient should be instructed to make sure to eat regular food to secure appropriate energy and protein intake. If there is any suggestion of a risk for malnutrition, poor intake, loss of appetite or any overt signs of poor nutritional status, nutritional supplements should be prescribed to the patient. These can be the regular supplements providing 1 kcal/mL, or supplements with 50% more energy and some extra protein. These should be taken daily along with the regular food, 400–800 mL per day [15]. Many patients about to undergo elective colorectal surgery consume too little energy and protein and are in a semi-starving state. There are several flavours and types of these supplements, and if there are any concerns with tastes, appetite or eating environment, it also advised to seek the consultation of a dietician in this phase [17].

In patients with overt nutritional problems, i.e., involuntary weight loss of more than 5% in the last 3 months or so, or even more recent changes such as rapid drop in food intake in the last couple of weeks, or overt clinical signs of malnutrition, more close attention to nutritional needs are warranted. Many cases can be handled as outpatients with the support of dieticians and nursing staff for ensuring the intake of food, supplements or enteral nutrition, but some will require hospital treatment with intravenous nutrition for up to 10 days to minimise the risks of the surgery [18, 19]. These include the patients that are unable to consume sufficient energy and protein via the enteral route. In many cases, this is a relative problem allowing a combination to be used. The enteral route is used for as much as it can take and the additional needs supplied with intravenous nutrition.

Physiological Effects of Bowel Preparation

Bowel preparation has been in use for decades before elective colorectal surgery. It was undertaken based on the belief that this step would reduce complications by minimising the risk of faecal content contaminating the perioneoal cavity and the wound. However, large randomised trials have shown that the use of mechanical bowel preparation before colonic surgery has no such protective effect. In fact it has no effect at all on outcome, as recently reviewed [20, 21]. It does however have major effects on hydration [20] and it stops the patient from having a meal in the afternoon and evening the day before surgery. This results in a prolonged period of fasting. This is not benefical for the patient, as outlined below. For colonic surgery, mechanical bowel prepartion should not be used routinely. For rectal surgery, the information available is less clear [21].

Preoperative Carbohydrates Instead of Overnight Fasting

Preoperative fasting was first proposed in 1848 after the first fatal anaesthesia [22], and became the dogma during the last century [23]. Despite overwhelming evidence for liberal fasting guidelines proposing intake of clear fluids up until 2 h before the onset of anaesthesia and surgery [24, 25], this ancient routine is still practised in many countries. In addition to causing unnecessary discomfort for the patients, the fasted state of metabolism coming in to surgical stress has been shown not to be optimal [26]. Instead of fasting, preparing the patient with a carbohydrate load has been shown to have several positive effects on outcomes after elective surgery. Many of these effects can be associated with the effect on insulin action and insulin sensitivity that a carbohydrate load can have.

The normal diurnal rhythm can be separated into two major entities: day-time metabolism that starts with breakfast and night-time metabolism that prevails during the later phase of the night. The two are very much influenced by insulin. When we eat breakfast, insulin is released and activates several mechanisms to ensure that the body stores the nutrients just consumed. Since digestion is slow and takes a few hours, the effects of insulin remain for several hours and are usually still active by the time the next meal is taken. This results in a day-time metabolism that is dominated by storage and anabolism under the influence of insulin. It is only during the night when the interval between meals is prolonged that the effects of insulin vanes, and other hormones prepare the body for the coming day. These hormones, mainly glucagon and cortisol, are both anti-insulin and catabolic and set metabolism in a breakdown mode. This is the situation that the body comes into surgery if in an overnight fasted state.

A 20% glucose infusion intravenously overnight or intake of 2–400 mL of a carbohydrate-rich drink at a concentration of around 12% has been used to break the overnight fasted state, set day-time metabolism and carbohydrate load to the patient. This initiates the activation of glucose uptake in insulin-sensitive organs (mainly muscle and fat) and breaks the overnight fasted and catabolic state before the surgery [27]. Intake of a carbohydrate-rich drink also enhances insulin sensitivity. This is likely to be one of the main reasons for the postoperative effect of substantially lower insulin resistance with the use of the carbohydrate treatment. This has effects mainly on the peripheral uptake of glucose in the first day or two [28, 29], while later the effects of a carbohydrate load is to reduce endogenous glucose production [30]. Both these effects will lower glucose levels, but in different ways. Interestingly, some of the effects remain for a very long time after surgery, as indicated by a report from Denmark showing that glycogen storage capacity was reduced in fasted patients up to a month after elective colorectal surgery while this was much improved with a preoperative carbohydrate load [31]. The mechanisms behind these effects on glucose and protein have recently become more clear with studies showing that the insulin signalling pathways for the major anabolic effects in muscle cells are better preserved with carbohydrate treatment compared to placebo [5]. This is likely to be due to the stimulation of these pathways before the onset of stress by the carbohydrate load.

Preoperative carbohydrates also affect other parts of metabolism. Thus, protein metabolism is better maintained [32, 33], lean body mass retained [34] and muscle function in the postoperative phase better maintained [31, 33]. Not just skeletal muscle is affected by metabolism and carbohydrate treatment, but also the cardiac muscle. Hence, several reports have shown that the heart functions better in carbohydrate-loaded state as opposed to fasted state [35–37]. These effects on muscle and the heart will impact on recovery in a positive way.

Epidural Anaesthesia and Analgesia

Part of the catabolic response is mediated by the release of adrenal hormones, cortisol and catecholamines. This release can effectively be blocked by the use of epidural anaesthesia [38]. The placement of the epidural should be such that it covers the dermatomes around Th10 for this effect. Importantly, this should be checked by activating the epidural before the onset of surgery to avoid the release of these potent catabolic hormones.

The epidural has several other effects that will be described elsewhere in more detail but one such effect that is related to the metabolic aspects of enhanced recovery is pain relief. It has very elegantly been shown that pain itself causes insulin resistance [39]. Thus avoiding pain is a key feature during the postoperative phase where the epidural plays a key role.

When combining the epidural with the carbohydrate treatment, thus addressing the insulin resistance in two different ways (as outlined above), a combined effect can be achieved. This was shown to allow complete enteral feeding to be given immediately after major colorectal surgery and continued for several days without any need of insulin to keep glucose levels within the normal range (6 mmol/L). This was achieved because the two treatments basically completely blocked the development of insulin resistance and the patient in a more balanced metabolic state was able to take care of glucose control with endogenous insulin release [40]. This is important since rigorous glucose control is difficult to achieve on regular surgical wards since it often require intravenous insulin that needs continuous adjustments.

Postoperative Nutrition and Metabolism

One of the main goals for enhanced recovery after surgery protocols is to have the patient back on oral intake as fast as possible, this being a key function necessary for discharge. To have the patient eating normally again necessitates two major goals to be met. The patient must tolerate the intake of food and the patient must be metabolically receptive to the nutrient given in order to make good use of them.

To have the patient tolerate normal food involves gut motility and appetite. Behind these functions lies also fluid balance and neural regulation of the gastrointestinal tract. This is being discussed elsewhere in more detail, while here the metabolic issue will be discussed.

As has been discussed above, hyperglycaemia is a key marker of surgical stress, and elevated glucose levels have been associated with a range of complications after surgery such as infections, neural problems, kidney failure, cardiac problems and muscle weakness. Some of these effects have been attributed or associated with the availability of carbohydrates inside muscle cells, such as the heart [36]. More recent studies show that preoperative carbohydrates impact postoperative signalling systems inside the cells to ensure a more anabolic function being retained. In addition, the epidural will further balance the stress responses by reducing the outflow of stress hormones and controlling pain. If feeding is pursued immediately after surgery and energy and protein goals are met, the starvation-induced catabolism is also avoided. By combining these treatments, the body metabolism can be maintained almost normal and this will render the patient a minimum of catabolism and an anabolic or at least balanced metabolism to support healing, control hyperglycaemia and minimize protein losses and muscle function.

How to Ensure Optimal Metabolism in Clinical Practice

Preoperative outpatient visit: During this visit, the decision to operate is usually taken. The patient will have to overcome the potential shock of the information of the fact that they have cancer and need an operation before they are given any further information. Hence this is often not the optimal time for detailed information about what the patient should do or how they best can participate in their own recovery. For this reason, it is best to focus on the patient's physical appearance – is this patient malnourished? Check for sign of malnutrition and order dietetic counselling and/or nutritional support. Decide if the patient can be nourished as an outpatient or if hospitalisation is needed. Control for any other metabolic problems, in particular diabetes. If so check glucose control and HbA1c to get insights into recent glucose control. Consider referral to an endocrinologist if glucose control is poor. The goal is to have the diabetic patient as anabolic as possible during the period before the operation.

Plan for a second visit for more detailed information where the patient and a relative/caretaker meet a nurse at the ward. This time it is important to involve the patient in their own recovery and one of the missions they will have is to both eat food and take the supplements after the operation. It is also worthwhile to introduce the supplements before the operation, so the patient can get used to them. At this time the patient should also be informed about the preoperative fasting regimen and the carbohydrate treatment.

Preoperative bowel preparation should be avoided. For most patients undergoing elective colonic resections bowel preparation is unnecessary. It has no beneficial effect on outcomes in colonic surgery [21], but will cause dehydration [20] and keep the patient from eating and thus set off a period of prolonged starvation. This will not be beneficial for the patient and should be avoided as much as possible. For rectal resections, the evidence is less clear and no clear recommendation can be made based on scientific evidence.

Preoperative fasting: Overnight fasting should only be used in selected cases where there is a known problem of gastric emptying or slow or impaired gastric motility that would represent a risk for aspiration. Except for certain diagnosis such as cancer in the upper gastro-intestinal tract, these cases are relatively rare, meaning that the overwhelming majority of patients about to undergo elective surgery can adhere to modern fasting guidelines [25]. These are: no solids for 6 h before anaesthesia and surgery, and recommend free intake of clear liquids until 2 h before anaesthesia and surgery.

Carbohydrate treatment: Carbohydrate treatment is recommended to all patients undergoing elective surgery in the most recent guidelines [25] with some caution for patients with diabetes. However, recent studies show that in well-controlled diabetic patients, gastric emptying is as fast as in healthy individuals [41]. If the patient is having bowel preparation the evening before the operation or for some other reason is not allowed to eat, an evening dose of 800 mL has been used for the 12.5% preparation of carbohydrates that has been most widely tested and used in clinical practice. All patients should have 400 mL as a morning dose to set metabolism before the operation. If the operation is planned for the afternoon, the patient can take 200 mL every hour up until 2 h before the operation. If it is a late afternoon operation, many patients can also have a regular breakfast given that a 6-h interval can be allowed for.

Epidural anaesthesia: An important aspect from a metabolic point of view is to have the epidural placed and activated before the onset of the operation. The 10th dermatome should be covered, and preferably also all the way up to the 4th dermatome to ensure blocking of adrenergic nerves to the pylorus that otherwise may slow down gastric emptying. Secondly, the epidural should stay in place and serve as the basic pain relief for at least 48 h. This will secure gastric motility by minimising the use of opioids and at the same time avoid pain causing insulin resistance.

Postoperative oral intake: As soon as the patient is lucid after the operation, she can be offered to drink clear fluids. After a couple of hours or so, intake of normal food can be allowed, and the patient should also take two cartons of nutritional supplements the same afternoon/evening of surgery. Preferably, eating and taking supplements can be done after getting out of bed after the operation, since this is the most normal way to eat or drink.

The day after surgery, the i.v. infusion should be disconnected in the morning. The patient should be served normal breakfast and from then on the hospital meals. On top of this they should be ordered two supplements with a total of at least 400 kcal a day. They should be instructed to drink as much as they want to, but at least 1,000 mL/day. Nursing staff should take notes on food and fluid intake daily and report any problems occurring.

In case of ileus or even vomiting, the intake should be stopped for a couple of hours and then resumed with fluids initially. If they work, the patient can start to eat again. If there is a suspicion of gastric retention, a nasogastric tube can be used to empty the contents. Once this is done, the tube should be removed and the patient starts to resume drinking within a couple of hours. The tube should not primarily stay in. Keeping a nasogastric tube in should be reserved for patients with an established ileus and for as short a period as possible (Table 3.1).

Table 3.1 Actions to take to minimize metabolic stress in ERAS protocols

When	Which patient	Action
Outpatient clinic	The undernourished patient	Oral supplements (if the gut is working)
		Dietary advice
		If not eating properly combine enteral and parenteral nutrition
	The patient who is slowly losing weight	Oral supplements and dietary advice
Day before surgery	Elective colon resections	Avoid bowel cleansing
	All	Eat normal hospital food
Before operation	All allowed to drink	Carbohydrate treatment 2 h before anaesthesia
	All	Thoracic epidural activated
Postoperatively day of surgery	All	As soon as the patient is lucid: propose clear fluids
		400 mL oral supplement
		Offer dinner
Day after surgery	All	Disconnect i.v. infusion in the morning after operation
		Breakfast, lunch and dinner offered
		2×200 mL oral supplements
		Free intake of fluids
		Secure good pain control

References

1. Thorell A, Nygren J, Ljungqvist O. Insulin resistance: a marker of surgical stress. Curr Opin Clin Nutr Metab Care. 1999;2(1):69–78.
2. Brandi LS et al. Insulin resistance after surgery: normalization by insulin treatment. Clin Sci (Lond). 1990;79(5):443–50.
3. Brownlee M. The pathobiology of diabetic complications: a unifying mechanism. Diabetes. 2005;54(6):1615–25.
4. Witasp A et al. Increased expression of inflammatory pathway genes in skeletal muscle during surgery. Clin Nutr. 2009;28(3):291–8.
5. Wang ZG et al. Randomized clinical trial to compare the effects of preoperative oral carbohydrate *versus* placebo on insulin resistance after colorectal surgery. Br J Surg. 2010;97(3):327–38.
6. Witasp A et al. Expression of inflammatory and insulin signaling genes in adipose tissue in response to elective surgery. J Clin Endocrinol Metab. 2010;95(7):3460–9.
7. Gore DC et al. Hyperglycemia exacerbates muscle protein catabolism in burn-injured patients. Crit Care Med. 2002;30(11):2438–42.
8. van den Berghe G et al. Intensive insulin therapy in the critically ill patients. N Engl J Med. 2001;345(19):1359–67.
9. Krinsley JS. Effect of an intensive glucose management protocol on the mortality of critically ill adult patients. Mayo Clin Proc. 2004;79(8):992–1000.
10. Gustafsson UO et al. Haemoglobin A1c as a predictor of postoperative hyperglycaemia and complications after major colorectal surgery. Br J Surg. 2009;96(11):1358–64.
11. Nygren J, Nair KS. Differential regulation of protein dynamics in splanchnic and skeletal muscle beds by insulin and amino acids in healthy human subjects. Diabetes. 2003;52(6): 1377–85.
12. Ferrando AA et al. A submaximal dose of insulin promotes net skeletal muscle protein synthesis in patients with severe burns. Ann Surg. 1999;229(1):11–8.
13. Pierre EJ et al. Effects of insulin on wound healing. J Trauma. 1998;44(2):342–5.
14. Schwegler I et al. Nutritional risk is a clinical predictor of postoperative mortality and morbidity in surgery for colorectal cancer. Br J Surg. 2010;97:92–7.
15. Smedley F et al. Randomized clinical trial of the effects of preoperative and postoperative oral nutritional supplements on clinical course and cost of care. Br J Surg. 2004;91(8):983–90.
16. Doenst T et al. Hyperglycemia during cardiopulmonary bypass is an independent risk factor for mortality in patients undergoing cardiac surgery. J Thorac Cardiovasc Surg. 2005; 130(4):1144.
17. Weimann A et al. ESPEN guidelines on enteral nutrition: surgery including organ transplantation. Clin Nutr. 2006;25(2):224–44.
18. Buzby GP et al. Perioperative totalparenteral nutrition in surgical patients. N Engl J Med. 1991;325:525–32.
19. Braga M et al. ESPEN Guidelines on Parenteral Nutrition: Surgery. Clin Nutr. 2009;28(4):378–86.
20. Holte K et al. Physiologic effects of bowel preparation. Dis Colon Rectum. 2004;47(8): 1397–402.
21. Slim K et al. Updated systematic reveiw and meta-analysis of randomized clincial trials on the role of mechanical bowel preparatyion before colorectal surgery. Ann Surg. 2009;249:203–9.
22. Fatal applications of chloroform. Section on legal medicine. Edinburgh Med J. 1848;69:498–503.
23. Maltby JR. Fasting from midnight - the history behind the dogma. Best Pract Res Clin Anaesthesiol. 2006;20(3):363–78.
24. Soreide E et al. Pre-operative fasting guidelines: an update. Acta Anaesthesiol Scand. 2005; 49(8):1041–7.

25. Powell-Tuck J et al. British consensus guidelines on intravenous fluid therapy for adult surgical patients. Journal of the Intensive Care Society. 2009;10(1):13–5.
26. Ljungqvist O. Modulating postoperative insulin resistance by preoperative carbohydrate treatment. Best Pract Res Clin Anaesthesiol. 2009;23:401–9.
27. Svanfeldt M et al. Effect of "preoperative" oral cardohydrate treatment on insulin action - a randomized cross-over unblinded study in healthy subjects. Clin Nutr. 2005;24:815–21.
28. Nygren J et al. Site of insulin resistance after surgery: the contribution of hypocaloric nutrition and bed rest. Clin Sci (Lond). 1997;93(2):137–46.
29. Soop M et al. Preoperative oral carbohydrate treatment attenuates immediate postoperative insulin resistance. Am J Physiol Endocrinol Metab. 2001;280(4):E576–83.
30. Soop M et al. Preoperative oral carbohydrate treatment attenuates endogenous glucose release 3 days after surgery. Clin Nutr. 2004;23(4):733–41.
31. Henriksen MG et al. Effects of preoperative oral carbohydrates and peptides on postoperative endocrine response, mobilization, nutrition and muscle function in abdominal surgery. Acta Anaesthesiol Scand. 2003;47(2):191–9.
32. Schricker T et al. Anticatabolic effects of avoiding preoperative fasting by intravenous hypocaloric nutrition: a randomized clinical trial. Ann Surg. 2008;248(6):1051–9.
33. Svanfeldt M et al. Randomized clinical trial of the effect of preoperative oral carbohydrate treatment on postoperative whole-body protein and glucose kinetics. Br J Surg. 2007;94(11):1342–50.
34. Yuill KA et al. The administration of an oral carbohydrate-containing fluid prior to major elective upper-gastrointestinal surgery preserves skeletal muscle mass postoperatively-a randomised clinical trial. Clin Nutr. 2005;24(1):32–7.
35. Oldfield GS, Commerford PJ, Opie LH. Effects of preoperative glucose-insulin-potassium on myocardial glycogen levels and on complications of mitral valve replacement. J Thorac Cardiovasc Surg. 1986;91(6):874–8.
36. Lolley DM et al. Clinical experience with preoperative myocardial nutrition management. J Cardiovasc Surg (Torino). 1985;26(3):236–43.
37. Breuer JP et al. Preoperative oral carbohydrate administration to ASA III-IV patients undergoing elective cardiac surgery. Anesth Analg. 2006;103(5):1099–108.
38. Uchida I et al. Effect of epidural analgesia on postoperative insulin resistance as evaluated by insulin clamp technique. Br J Surg. 1988;75(6):557–62.
39. Greisen J et al. Acute pain induces insulin resistance in humans. Anesthesiology. 2001;95(3):578–84.
40. Soop M et al. Randomized clinical trial of the effects of immediate enteral nutrition on metabolic responses to major colorectal surgery in an enhanced recovery protocol. Br J Surg. 2004;91:1138–45.
41. Gustafsson UO et al. Pre-operative carbohydrate treatment may be used in type 2 diabetes patients. Acta Anaesthesiol Scand. 2008;52(7):946–51.

Chapter 4
Anaesthetic Contributions in Enhanced Recovery

Monty G. Mythen and Michael Scott

Introduction

Enhanced recovery (ER) not only reduces length of stay in hospital for patients but can help reduce the development of complications. The development of a complication during major surgery has important implications for patients beyond that of immediate morbidity and mortality risk. In 2005 Khuri and colleagues published a study from a database of 105,951 patients undergoing eight common operations. It showed the key determinant of reduced postoperative survival at follow-up at 8 years was the occurrence of a complication within 30 days of surgery. Rapid recovery without complications after surgery may also offer survival benefits for cancer patients because patients are fitter sooner after surgery to have follow on chemotherapy.

The anaesthetist must therefore use available evidence-based techniques and drug therapy to reduce the number of complications after surgery. Patients who are more likely to develop a complication during the peri-operative period should be identified at pre-assessment. Pre-existing medical problems should be optimised such as anaemia, pulmonary and cardiac function. Ideally if time permits the patients should have their own exercise programme to improve fitness prior to surgery. Finally the patient is placed on the correct care pathway to ensure optimal management.

M.G. Mythen
Centre for Anaesthesia, University College of London, London, UK

M. Scott (✉)
Department of Anaesthetics and Intensive Care Medicine, Royal Surrey County
NHS Foundation Trust, University of Surrey, Guildford, Surrey, UK

N. Francis et al. (eds.), *Manual of Fast Track Recovery for Colorectal Surgery*,
Enhanced Recovery, DOI 10.1007/978-0-85729-953-6_4,
© Springer-Verlag London Limited 2012

The Role of the Anaesthetist

1. Identification and optimising the patient's co-morbidities prior to surgery.
2. Reducing the patient's peri-operative risk using available evidence-based techniques and drug therapy.
3. Delivering a modern anaesthetic technique to minimise postoperative nausea and vomiting to enable early gut function.
4. To provide effective analgesia using regional anaesthetic techniques combined with multimodal analgesia to enable early feeding and mobility.
5. Peri-operative individualised goal-directed fluid therapy
6. Minimising secondary complications such as thromboembolic disease, wound and chest infection.

Pre-assessment Identification of Patients with Reduced Functional Capacity, Increased Cardiovascular Risk and Optimisation

Patients presenting for elective major surgery should be assessed in a specific anaesthetic lead preoperative assessment clinic as an outpatient prior to coming to hospital for surgery. At this visit anaesthesia and the ER programme can be explained. Some units use this visit to meet the ER nurse specialist and stoma care nurse as well and then obtaining informed consent from the patient.

Clinical examination together with baseline investigations such as full blood count, urea and electrolytes, liver function tests, lung function tests and resting ECG can provide further information. MRSA screening can be done at this point.

Each patient should have:

1. Functional capacity assessed
2. Their cardiovascular risk index determined
3. Optimisation of any health problems
4. Commencement of beta-blockers or statins if indicated

Risk Factors for Major Surgery

1. *Age*: Increasing age is a risk factor for surgery.
2. *Type of surgery*: The type of surgery the patient has performed has different risks of MI and cardiac death within 30 days. These have been classified by Boersma et al. [1] . (Fig. 4.1).

Low –risk < 1%	Intermediate-risk 1-5%	High-risk > 5%
Breast	Abdominal	Aortic and major vascular surgery
Dental	Carotid	Peripheral vascular surgery
Endocrine	Peripheral arterial angioplasty	
Eye	Endovascular aneurysm repair	
Gynaecology	Head and neck surgery	
Reconstructive	Neurological /orthopaedic – major (hip and spine surgery)	
Orthopaedic – minor (knee surgery)	Pulmonary renal / liver transplant	
Urological - minor	Urological - major	

Fig. 4.1   Surgical risk estimate as described by Boersma et al.

Functional Capacity

Estimating functional capacity is an important start of assessing a patient. Functional capacity is measured in metabolic equivalents (METs). One MET equals the basal metabolic rate at rest. Climbing two flights of stairs demands 4 METs and strenuous activity playing sport or swimming is >10 METS. The inability to perform 4 METS indicates poor functional capacity and is associated with an increased incidence of postoperative cardiac events. The presence of good functional capacity, even in the presence of stable ischaemic heart disease (IHD) or other risk factors is associated with a good outcome [2].

Cardiac Risk Index in Non-cardiac Surgery: The Lee Index

In 1999 Lee and colleagues described the Lee index, which is a modification of the original Goldman index. The Lee index contains five independent clinical determinants of major peri-operative cardiac events:

1. History of IHD
2. History of cerebrovascular disease
3. Heart failure
4. Insulin-dependent diabetes mellitus
5. Impaired renal function
6. High-risk type of surgery

All factors contribute 1 point equally to the index, and for patients with an index of 0, 1, 2, and 3 points the incidence of major cardiac complications is estimated at 0.4%, 0.9%, 7%, and 11%, respectively.

Table 4.1 Active cardiac conditions for which the patient should undergo evaluation and treatment before noncardiac surgery (Class I, Level of Evidence: B)

Condition examples	
Unstable coronary syndromes	Unstable or severe angina[a] (CCS class III or IV)[b]
	Recent MI[c]
Decompensated HF (NYHA functional class IV; worsening or new-onset HF)	
Significant arrhythmias	High-grade atrioventricular block
	Mobitz II atrioventricular block
	Third-degree atrioventricular heart block
	Symptomatic ventricular arrhythmias
	Supraventricular arrhythmias (including atrial fibrillation) with uncontrolled ventricular rate (HR greater than 100 bpm at rest)
	Symptomatic bradycardia
	Newly recognised ventricular tachycardia
Severe valvular disease	Severe aortic stenosis (mean pressure gradient greater than 40 mmHg aortic valve area less than 1.0 cm^2, or symptomatic)
	Symptomatic mitral stenosis (progressive dyspnoea on exertion, exertional presyncope, or HF)

CCS Canadian Cardiovascular Society, HF heart failure, HR heart rate, MI myocardial infarction, NYHA New York Heart Association
[a]According to Campeau.10
[b]May include stable angina in patients who are unusually sedentary
[c]The American College of Cardiology National Database Library defines recent MI as more than 7 days but less than or equal to 1 month (within 30 days)

The need for further evaluation and treatment before surgery for patients who have heart problems can be obtained by referring to the American Heart Association (AHA) guidelines (Table 4.1).

South Devon healthcare Trust has successfully devised a preoperative assessment tool to triage patients according to risk of mortality and morbidity specifically for elective hip and knee replacement combining age, functional capacity, cardiovascular risk factors and surgery. It uses a traffic light system to determine who performs the preoperative assessment and whether the patients undergoes cardiopulmonary (CPX) testing (Fig. 4.2).

Assessing Cardiopulmonary Status Using Cardiopulmonary Exercise Testing

Cardiopulmonary exercise testing (CPET) is a dynamic non-invasive objective test that evaluates the ability of a patient's cardiopulmonary system to adapt to a sudden increase in oxygen demand. The ramped exercise test is performed on a cycle ergometer. With increasing exercise, oxygen consumption will eventually exceed oxygen

Preoperative assessment: Triage			
Risk	**1**	**2**	**3**
Age	<78	78–82	>82
IHD		Angina (no MI)	MI/NSTEMI
Heart failure		Heart failure	
Creatinine	<90 µmol/L	91–149 µmol/L	>150 µmol/L
TIA/stroke		One TIA	Two TIAs or one stroke
Diabetes		NIDDM	IDDM
Short of breath		SOB	
Confusion		Confusion	
CABG or Stents		CABG or Stents	
PE		PE	
Previous problem		Previous problem	
Malignancy		Malignancy	
Patient request		Patient request	
Worried		Worried	
Falls		Falls	
Revision surgery		Revision surgery	
Bilateral surgery		Bilateral surgery	
Assessment by	Nurse	Nurse + Anaesthetist	Anaesthetist – CPX

Creatinine Look for current and previous blood results. If raised in past use highest measurement
TIA/CVA Transient ischaemic attach or cerebrovascular accident
Diabetes Consider duration of diabetes, control of blood sugar and other organ damage
Short of breath Shortness at breath at rest or minimal exercise
Confusion Currently confused or history of confusion or dementia
Previous problem During previous admission that may recur
Worried Any concern that needs discussion
CPX Cardiopulmonary exercise

Source: South Devon Healthcare NHS Trust – model based on the peri-operative risk for elective hip and knee replacement

Fig. 4.2 South Devon Healthcare Trust's triage system for preoperative assessment – elective hip and knee replacement (Source: South Devon Healthcare NHS Trust – model based on the peri-operative risk for elective hip and knee replacement)

delivery. Aerobic metabolism becomes inadequate to meet the metabolic demands and blood lactate rises, reflecting supplementary anaerobic metabolism. The value for oxygen consumption at this point is known as the anaerobic threshold (AT), expressed as mL/kg/min. Original work by Older has shown a greater mortality in patients with an AT below 11 mL/kg/min undergoing major abdominal surgery, the risk being compounded by the presence of IHD [3, 4]. More recent work by Snowden and colleagues has shown an increase in postoperative complications and length of stay in hospital in patients with submaximal cardiopulmonary exercise testing. The study showed that CPET was more sensitive a predictor than the preoperative activity questionnaire patients completed. An AT of 10.1 mL/kg/min or greater in this group of patients predicted a lower risk of complications [5]. The VO_2 max achieved during CPET has also been shown to be an important variable to measure outcome for major surgery but more so if the patient is undergoing thoracic surgery.

Optimisation of Pre-existing Disease

Patients with pre-existing pulmonary and cardiac disease should have their conditions optimised by their GP or physician. Anaemia should be screened for, detected and corrected before admission for surgery. Cessation of smoking should be encouraged.

Cardiovascular Risk Reduction

There has been much focus on beta-blockers and statins to reduce peri-operative myocardial ischaemic events and peri-operative myocardial infarction. The following are the Class 1 evidence-based AHA recommendations [6]:

(a) Statins: Class 1 Recommendations

- Statins should be started in high-risk patients, optimally between 30 days and at least 1 week before surgery (Class 1 B).
- Statins should be continued peri-operatively (Class 1 C).

(b) Beta Blockers: Class 1 Recommendations

- Beta-blockers are recommended in patients who have known IHD or myocardial ischaemia according to preoperative stress testing (Class 1 B).
- Beta-blockers are recommended in patients scheduled for high-risk surgery (Class 1 B) (30 days, at least 1 week prior to surgery. *Target HR 60–70*, systolic BP>100 mmHg).
- Continuation of beta-blockers is recommended in patients previously treated with beta-blockers because of IHD, arrhythmias or hypertension (Class 1 C).

Specific Drugs Which Are Important to Identify Preoperatively

Certain drugs should be identified preoperatively as they require special management through the peri-operative period and if not managed correctly can increase the risk of peri-operative complications:

1. Aspirin – follow local hospital policy
2. Clopidogrel with coronary stent – liaise with the patient's cardiologist
3. Warfarin – liaise with the patient's haematologist
4. ACE inhibitors – consider omitting on morning of surgery

Simplifying the Anaesthetic Approach to Delivering Enhanced Recovery

In 2007 Scott and Fawcett simplified the 20 key elements of enhanced recovery into a trimodal approach for the anaesthetist. They separated out the two key areas that an anaesthetist has control over: fluid therapy and analgesia and delivered the other elements of ER via a protocol-based enhanced recovery pathway (see Fig. 4.3). In 2009 Levy Scott Fawcett and Rockal combined these key elements using carefully delivered spinal anaesthesia combined with general anaesthesia to produce the first series of 23-h stay for colorectal resection within a randomised controlled trial [7].

Fig. 4.3 A simplified trimodal approach for anaesthetists described by Scott and Fawcett delivers the non-surgical components of ER using a protocol-based ER pathway. The two remaining elements of fluid therapy and analgesia are extremely important in effecting outcome for which the anaesthetist is responsible

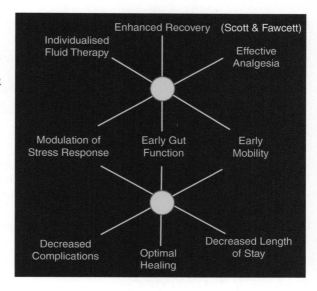

The enhanced recovery elements help to normalise patient's physiology and homeostasis. Individualised fluid therapy using stroke volume optimisation ensures that global oxygen delivery and hepato-splanchnic blood supply is optimised. At the same time avoidance of liberal amounts of salt containing fluid in the postoperative period reduces gut ileus and encourages return of gut function and early feeding. The use of regional analgesia during surgery helps modulate the stress response and reduce gut ileus. Early enteral feeding can help change the patient's catabolic response to surgery to anabolic and this promotes healing. Early mobility and healing with return to normal body homeostasis decreases complications, which in turn lead to decreased length of stay.

Day of Surgery

Admission to Hospital and Preoperative Preparation

- Same day admission is preferred by patients as they sleep better the night before surgery in their own bed. It also improves utilisation of beds in the hospital.
- Premedication with sedatives or anxiolytics should be avoided if possible.
- The duration of fasting should be 6 h for solids and 2 h for liquids.
- Carbohydrate drinks the night before surgery and up to 2 h before surgery improves patient's well-being, reduces dehydration and reduces insulin resistance during major surgery.

Conduct of Anaesthesia

- Standard preoperative checks, e.g. World Health Organisation Surgical Safety Checklist.
- Full monitoring and large bore intravenous access established.
- Regional anaesthetic block plus test dose if needed.
- Induction with propofol and a short-acting opioid.
- Short-acting non-depolarising muscle relaxant is used to facilitate intubation and ventilation.
- Maintenance of anaesthesia – short-acting volatile agents or target-controlled intravenous propofol infusions with oxygen-enriched air.
- Avoid nitrous oxide because of its effects on the bowel and increase risk of nausea and vomiting.
- Remifentanil infusion or short-acting opioids as needed.

Nasogastric Tubes in GI Surgery

- Can impair return of gut function.
- Are disliked by patients.
- Increase the incidence of postoperative fever, atelectasis and pneumonia.
- Lower GI surgery: Only insert if gastric distension or requested by surgeon.
- Upper GI Surgery: May be necessary.

Anti-microbial Prophylaxis

- Antibiotic prophylaxis has been shown to reduce the risk of infective complications in surgery [8].
- The local hospital antibiotic policy should be followed.
- Optimum timing in colorectal surgery has been shown to be 1 h before skin incision.
- If operations last more than 3 h a further dose of antibiotics should be administered [8].

Urinary Drainage

- Aim to remove urinary catheters the morning after surgery.
- The risk of urinary retention after colonic resection above the peritoneal reflection after 24 h is low, even if low concentration dose epidural analgesia is used [9].
- Catheterisation may need to be continued if the patient has problems with voiding due to surgical or other physiological issues.

- A recent meta-analysis showed that suprapubic catheterisation may be more acceptable for patients and associated with lower morbidity when used in pelvic operations [10].

Avoiding Peri-operative Hypothermia

- Warm air blowers on the patients during surgery.
- Warm intravenous fluids administered.
- Warming should be continued into the postoperative period [11].
- Temperature monitoring is mandatory to guide warming and also avoid hyperthermia.
- Hypothermia increases the risk of wound infection, bleeding and transfusion requirements [12, 13].
- Maintaining the temperature above 36.7°C may also reduce the risk of morbid cardiac events [14].

Prevention of Postoperative Nausea and Vomiting (PONV)

- PONV has a major impact on patient recovery.
- PONV is unpleasant, delays gut function, affects mobility and has metabolic consequences.
- All patients should receive prophylactic anti-emetics during anaesthesia around 30 min before the end of surgery. A serotonin receptor antagonists such as ondansetron combined, as necessary, with an antihistamine such as cyclizine can be effective.
- Use a scoring system, e.g. Apfel's prediction model, to identify those patients at high risk of PONV: females, non-smokers, a history of motion sickness and post-operative opioid administration [15] are risk factors. Three or more factors predict a high risk of PONV and additional measures such as target-controlled propofol infusion to maintain anaesthesia ± single doses of dexamethasone may be necessary.
- It is unclear how dexamethasone effects the stress and metabolic response during major surgery – lowest effective dose, caution in diabetics.
- Droperidol in doses of 0.0625–1.25 mg is effective if morphine is used as the postoperative analgesic regime [16].

Monitoring and Vascular Access During Surgery

- Standard monitoring: ECG, pulse oximeter, non-invasive blood pressure, end tidal carbon dioxide (Et CO_2) and inspired anaesthetic gases and oxygen concentration
- Temperature monitoring
- Peripheral IV fluids given through a warming device

Arterial Pressure Monitoring

- Provides beat to beat heart rate, blood pressure and waveform.
- Arterial blood gases and blood loss.
- Useful in patients with cardiopulmonary disease who are more likely to have perioperative problems.
- Necessary if pulse contour wave analysis is being used.

Central Venous Lines and Monitoring

- Still commonly used during open major surgery.
- Complications reduced by using a sterile technique and ultrasound to locate the internal jugular vein during insertion.
- Multi-lumen central venous catheter provides excellent intravenous access in patients who have cardiopulmonary problems and those patients that may need vasopressor or inotrope infusions.
- Flow-directed monitoring has been shown to be superior to central venous pressure, which can often have very high values during laparoscopic procedures, hence why central venous lines insertion is losing favour to flow-directed fluid therapy techniques.

Individualised Goal-Directed Fluid Therapy: Fluid Therapy, Stroke Volume Optimisation and Oxygen Delivery

Peri-operative fluid therapy is one of the most important things that anaesthetists control that can affect outcome of the surgery. Fluids are discussed elsewhere in detail and hence covered here in brief. Evidence-based practice shows that there are several important strategies that can affect outcome from surgery related to fluid therapy.

Avoid Fluid Shifts

- Avoid bowel prep
- Avoid dehydration: Oral fluid/carbohydrate drink up to 2 h before surgery
- Reduction of bowel handling: Laparoscopic or laparoscopic-assisted surgery

Individualised Goal-Directed Fluids

- Stroke volume optimisation during surgery
- Measuring oxygen delivery during surgery $(DO_2)_i$ and increasing it if it is low

Postoperative Fluids

- Restrict salt and i.v. fluids while maintaining normovolaemia
- Encourage early enteral feeding

Stroke Volume Optimisation

Several studies have shown an improvement in outcome using stroke volume optimisation using oesophageal Doppler monitoring in major surgery [17, 18] and others specifically in colorectal surgery [19–21]. In all these studies it is interesting that stroke volume optimisation with fluids alone, without the measurement or targeting of oxygen delivery improves outcome. An extra bolus of 250 mL of fluid can be all that is necessary to optimise stroke volume and improve oxygen delivery.

Technique of Fluid Optimisation

The method of fluid optimisation described below was first described by Mythen [17] and has been used and adapted in many of the major studies which have shown an improvement in outcome using oesophageal Doppler [18–20]. A fluid challenge is given rapidly and the response in stroke volume observed. It is important to wait for 5 min after the fluid bolus before interpreting the change in stroke volume as it takes time for the circulation to adapt to these fluid boluses. Fluid boluses are repeated until the increase in stroke volume is less than 10% following the bolus. After time or if there is bleeding, the stroke volume will fall by 10% and a further fluid bolus is given (Fig. 4.4).

Timing of Stroke Volume Optimisation

It is important to optimise stroke volume before there are any major effects on the patient's circulation. These include putting the patient in a head up or down position, before their legs are put up in the Lloyd Davies position and preferably before any vasoconstrictors are commenced. At the end of surgery when the surgeon is suturing the skin there is a further opportunity to optimise stroke volume prior to waking the patient up and going to recovery.

Monitoring Cardiac Output and Oxygen Delivery

There are an increasing number of options for anaesthetists to use to measure cardiac output during anaesthesia. Each has advantages and disadvantages; however,

Fig. 4.4 Mythen's method of optimising stroke volume using colloid fluid boluses has been shown to improve outcome in major surgery in several randomised controlled studies

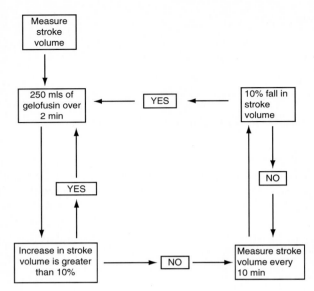

oesophageal Doppler monitoring is the only technology to have been validated in randomised controlled studies. Most of the devices can be utilised to optimise stroke volume and then calculate cardiac output and oxygen delivery for the patient (Fig. 4.5).

1. Oesophageal Doppler
2. Arterial waveform analysis; pulse power and pulse contour wave analysis

LIDCO Rapid® is a new portable monitor designed for theatre use. It utilises the LIDCO Plus® pulse power algorithm but without using lithium to calibrate it. A nomogram of the patient's age, height and weight is used to generate a nominal stroke volume (Fig. 4.6).

Oxygen Delivery and Goal-Directed Therapy

Every patient will have different oxygen requirements during surgery depending on their own physical and physiological variables, the extent of surgery and metabolic response to injury.

Oxygen delivery is usually expressed as a value per metre squared of body surface area. It is a product of the haemoglobin level × cardiac output × arterial oxygen saturation × 1.34:

- $DO_2I = Hb$ (g/l) × CO (l/min) × 1.34 × SaO_2/SA (m²)

Fig. 4.5 The Cardio Q® oesophageal Doppler machine is a simple non-invasive way of optimising stroke volume in patients during surgery

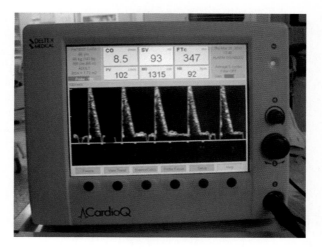

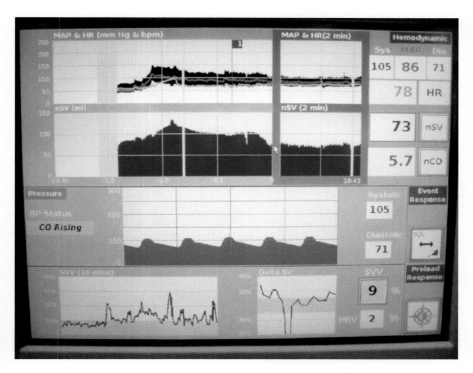

Fig. 4.6 The LIDCO Rapid® is a portable machine that can be used in the operating theatre. It works off the arterial waveform using pulse power analysis similar to LIDCO Plus but scaled based around a nomogram of the patient's age, height and weight to generate a nominal stroke volume

In 2005 Pearse showed that postoperative goal-directed therapy (GDT) to attain a target of an oxygen delivery index of 600 mL/min/m^2 was associated with a reduction in postoperative complications and duration of hospital stay. However, the patients in this study were not fluid optimised during surgery so it is unclear if the benefits seen in this study will be as great in elective surgical patients who have stroke volume optimisation during surgery. Further studies are needed to establish optimum oxygen delivery targets for different types of surgery, however patients identified as having a low oxygen delivery on table should be considered for postoperative optimisation using fluids and inotropes to reduce postoperative complications.

Which Fluids?

There continues to be controversy over which fluids to use in major surgery. Currently there is no clear evidence to support the use of colloids over crystalloid or vice versa; however, the studies that have used oesophageal Doppler to optimise stroke volume have all used fluid boluses using colloids to target stroke volume with postoperative fluids being crystalloid. The GIFTASUP guidelines recommend balanced salt solutions over normal saline. Once the patient is fluid optimised at the end of surgery there is no need to keep giving large quantities of salt containing intravenous fluid but normovolaemia should be maintained. Once enteral feeding is established the i.v. fluid should be stopped.

Analgesia

Analgesia is discussed in detail in Chap. 6.
   Analgesic methods should:

- Be effective and allow early mobilisation
- Avoid or reduce the amount of parenteral opioids given to the patient
- Utilise regional or local anaesthetic nerve blocks as appropriate
- Regular paracetamol and non-steroidal anti-inflammatory agents reduce the need/requirement of opioids

   Regional blocks

- Help modulate the stress response to surgery
- Increase oxygen delivery during surgery due to sympathetic block causing vasodilatation
- Can improve return of gut function by avoiding opioids
- Can cause postoperative hypotension

- Can reduce postoperative mobility if patients are not aided appropriately
- Can lead to increased postoperative intravenous fluid volumes being given

Modulation of the Stress Response

The stress response to surgery is complex and involves many pathways. Although a lot of emphasis traditionally is put on reducing the stress response it is clear that there are evolutionary reasons why humans have a stress response. We therefore discuss modulation of the stress response rather than obtunding it as some form of healing response is necessary and unavoidable due to local inflammatory effects. The factors that are part of the enhanced recovery pathway that help modulate the stress response fall into several groups but it is the sum of these that is important in a patient making an early recovery and feeling of well-being:

- Fluid therapy and avoidance of preoperative dehydration
- Early postoperative nutrition and avoidance of starvation
- Optimal analgesia and the use of a regional anaesthetic blockade during surgery
- Avoidance of nasogastric tubes, drains, prolonged urinary or central venous catheterisation, all of which can affect normal body physiology and homeostasis

Intraoperative Issues for the Anaesthetist

Comparing Open and Laparoscopic Surgery

Positioning of the Patient on the Operating Table

Open Surgery

For right-sided colonic operations patients are usually positioned supine. For pelvic, low anterior resections and left-sided colonic surgery the patient is positioned in the Lloyd Davies position to allow surgical access to the rectum. The patient's legs are put in a raised position using a suitable device such as Yellowfiins®. These take the pressure off the patient's calves. The use of flowtron boots in the Lloyd Davies position has been associated with compartment syndrome if the patient is head down for a period of time, so care must be taken to avoid this.

Laparoscopic Surgery

During laparoscopic resections the patient is often positioned with left or right lateral tilt combined with a steep head down position for pelvic surgery. It is imperative to

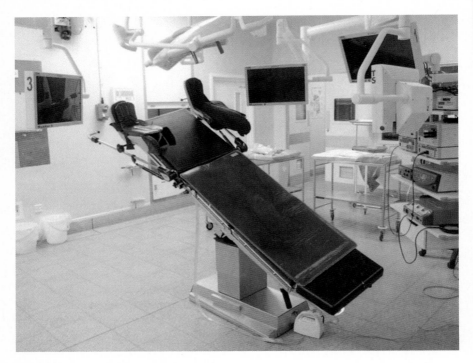

Fig. 4.7 The steep head down position necessary for laparoscopic colorectal surgery combined with a CO_2 pneumoperitoneum creates physiological stresses for the patient's cardiopulmonary system

carefully position the patient and wrap the arms and put jelly padding on any areas likely to be subject to pressure effect as the patient may be in this position for a prolonged period of time. Yellowfiins® can increase stability of the patient's position because they support and hold the legs in position. Any sliding sheets used to transfer the patient should be removed and the use of shoulder supports can stop the patient sliding down the operating table. The steep head down position as shown in Fig. 4.7 has marked effects on the patient's physiology, particularly when combined with insufflation of the peritoneum. These effects are discussed in more detail below.

Physiological Consequences of Surgery

Open Surgery

Open surgery has several disadvantages compared with laparoscopic surgery. There is more tissue damage, which can lead to a greater stress and systemic inflammatory response (SIRS). The gut is more likely to get an ileus because of bowel handling intra-operatively and fluid shifts postoperatively. Mobility after surgery can also be impaired. Carefully practised epidural analgesia can improve mobility and gut function after open surgery.

Laparoscopic Surgery

Despite the increasing adoption of laparoscopic techniques for major surgery, there has been surprisingly little published to date regarding the physiological consequences of establishing and maintaining a pneumoperitoneum.

Physiological Effects of Establishing a CO_2 Pneumoperitoneum

The physiological changes as a result of establishing a CO_2 pneumoperitoneum can affect many organs. The cardiorespiratory and fluid status of the patient has a major effect on the magnitude of these effects, as does positioning of the patient, particularly the steep head down/Trendelenberg position used in laparoscopic colorectal surgery [22].

Cardiovascular Effects

At insufflation there is a rapid rise in arterial blood pressure due to increase in aortic afterload [23]. Early work in laparoscopic surgery suggested a decrease in cardiac output at the time of insufflation due to a decrease in venous return. However, more recent work in fluid-optimised patients have shown that venous return is not as effected and may even increase [22, 24]. The increase in afterload has the effect of decreasing stroke volume. Work by Levy, Scott et al. showed that in fluid-optimised patients this increase in afterload is sustained for around 20–25 min and follows a similar pattern whether the patient has a regional block or not [25]. After this time the systemic vascular resistance drifts back to more normal levels. There is an increase in both left and right ventricular filling pressures and elevation of pulmonary pressures and vascular resistance [26]. Changing ventilator parameters and increasing PEEP with the resultant increase in mean airway pressure may expose the right ventricle to particularly high workload. Increases in right ventricular workload have also been demonstrated in transoesophageal echocardiography due to ventilation and CO_2 pneumoperitoneum [27]. In the head down position, care should therefore be exercised if changing ventilator parameters to increase mean airway intra-thoracic pressures as this will worsen right ventricular work.

Pulmonary Effects

During a CO_2 pneumoperitoneum there is increased abdominal wall compliance and reduction of lung volume due to the pressure exerted on the diaphragm. Respiratory mechanics are disrupted with less excursion of the diaphragm. Ventilation pressures therefore need to be increased to achieve the same tidal volumes before insufflation.

Renal Effects

The CO_2 pneumoperitoneum, patient positioning and duration of pneumoperitoneum all have compounding effects to reduce both renal blood flow and postoperative renal function [28]. Particular care should therefore be taken with patients with pre-existing renal dysfunction and insulin-dependent diabetics.

Complications of a Prolonged CO_2 Pneumoperitoneum in the Head Down Position

It is being increasingly recognised that very long laparoscopic procedures (>3.5–4 h) with the patient in the head down position can cause problems that do not occur during open surgery. The steep head down position and pneumoperitoneum can lead to venous engorgement of the head due to reduction in venous return. If arterial CO_2 rises then this is accompanied by a rise in cerebral blood flow, which can further exacerbate the problem [29]. This may lead to confusion and altered conscious level in the patient postoperatively and there have been reports of patients requiring ventilation postoperatively in order to control intracranial pressure due to the cerebral oedema.

Ventilation Strategy During Surgery

Ventilation strategy during surgery is aimed at maintaining an adequate arterial pO_2 and controlling pCO_2. It is also important to avoid barotrauma to the lungs secondary to high airway pressures and lung volumes.

Open Surgery

Ventilation during open surgery is usually straightforward unless the patient has severe cardiorespiratory co-morbidities; however, the ventilation of the lungs during laparoscopic surgery is not always straightforward. The level of PEEP is set to optimise functional residual capacity. The use of 'optimal' PEEP can be guided by flow volume loops. The tidal volume is adjusted using the peak inspiratory pressure so that together with the respiratory rate the target alveolar minute volume is achieved to maintain the required arterial pCO_2.

Laparoscopic Surgery

Ventilation during laparoscopic surgery can be challenging. In the steep head down position the peak airway pressure needed to achieve an adequate tidal volume can be high due to pneumoperitoneum and chest wall compliance. Although PEEP restores the functional residual capacity (FRC) combined with high inspiratory pressures the significant increase in mean airway pressure can lead to an increase in right ventricular stroke work. Pressure-controlled ventilation may be preferred and a higher ventilation rate but lower tidal lung volume (similar to a protective lung strategy model for acute lung injury).

Summary

Minimally invasive surgery has the potential to deliver postoperative benefits of improved mobility, reduced fluid shifts, reduced gut ileus, improved early gut function, reduced analgesic requirements and reduced SIRS response. However there are significant cardiopulmonary stresses for the patient during surgery which may be greater in certain circumstances than open surgery (Table 4.2).

Postoperative Care

Most patients can be discharged from the recovery area to a ward environment. Certain groups of patients should be considered for postoperative monitoring to include flow-directed studies to enable targeted oxygen delivery for 12 h. These include:

(a) Patients who have been identified preoperatively as having limited cardiopulmonary reserve
(b) Patients who at preoperative cardiopulmonary testing has demonstrated an anaerobic threshold of less than 10
(c) Patients who after stroke volume optimisation during surgery have an unexpectedly low oxygen delivery

Table 4.2 Summary of key physiological differences comparing laparoscopic and open major surgery

	Laparoscopic surgery	Open surgery
Cardiovascular risk	Equal to open surgery	Equal to laparoscopic surgery
Oxygen delivery	Can be reduced compared to open surgery due to increased aortic afterload and head down position	Can be increased during surgery due to epidural block
Ventilation	Can be impaired	Straightforward
Pain after surgery	Severe pain settles after 12–24 h so can be addressed with oral analgesia	Severe pain lasting up to 72 h
Fluid shifts	Minimised after 24 h unless gut ileus	Up to 72 h postoperatively.
Postoperative fluid requirements	Intravenous fluid rarely needed beyond 24 h	Intravenous fluids often carried on for duration of epidural
SIRS response	Reduced compared to open surgery	Substantial due to surgical wound and bowel handling
Gut ileus	Shorter – possibly due to there not being bowel handling	Can be prolonged
Renal function	Renal perfusion reduced significantly during surgery	Renal perfusion reduced
Mobility after surgery	Good	Impaired
Lung function after surgery	Improved compared to open surgery	Can be impaired if there is pre-existing pulmonary disease or inadequate analgesia

The first 12 h postoperatively is important in determining cellular response to injury and the healing process and careful management during this time may decrease the incidence of complications.

Preventing Secondary Complications

Reducing the Risk of Postoperative Chest Infection

During Surgery

Microaspiration into the lungs during surgery may contribute to postoperative chest infection.

Ways to protect against microaspiration include:

- PU cuffs on et tubes (Sealguard™, Taperguard™)
- PEEP
- Glycopyrronium
- Subglottic suctioning
- Awake extubation

Table 4.3 Risk factors for venous thromboembolism

Active cancer or cancer treatment
• Age over 60 years
• Critical care admission
• Dehydration
• Known thrombophilias
• Obesity (body mass index [BMI] over 30 kg/m²)
• One or more significant medical co-morbidities (e.g., heart disease; metabolic, endocrine or respiratory pathologies; acute infectious diseases; inflammatory conditions)
• Personal history or first-degree relative with a history of VTE
• Use of hormone replacement therapy
• Use of oestrogen-containing contraceptive therapy
• Varicose veins with phlebitis

Postoperatively

Postoperative lung function is improved by good analgesia, position and mobility. Levy et al. showed that there were only small differences in lung function (PEFR and FEV_1) in patients with or without a regional block undergoing laparoscopic surgery with all groups having a reduction in function [30]. In open surgery pulmonary function is improved with epidural analgesia. Patients should be nursed sitting upright or in a chair whenever possible because lying flat has a significant effect on the FRC of the lungs and respiratory muscle function. Increasing mobility and early walking is the most effective way of improving lung function. If patients are unable to mobilise early then incentive spirometry may be beneficial.

Preventing Venous Thromboembolism

The risk of venous thromboembolism (VTE) is not just during the peri-operative period but can last several weeks into the postoperative period after the patient has gone home. The causes of thromboembolism are multifactorial and additive. Each patient should have an individual risk score calculated before surgery and suitable precautions implemented according to local or national guidelines (Table 4.3).

Prevention

Measures to decrease the risk of venous thromboembolism:

- Maintaining hydration
- Early mobilisation

- Surgical compression stockings, e.g. TEDs™ prior to surgery, and these should be worn during their stay in hospital.
- Fractionated heparin and subcutaneous low molecular weight heparin (LMWH). Studies have shown both to be effective in reducing deep vein thrombosis (DVT), pulmonary embolism (PE) and mortality in patients undergoing colorectal surgery [31–34].
- Meta-analyses have shown that there to be no difference in efficacy or bleeding risks between LMWH and unfractionated heparin; however, LMWH appears to be preferred due to its once-daily dosing.
- The use of LMWH impacts the way that epidural analgesia can be practiced by the anaesthetist. There is an increased risk of epidural haematoma if epidural catheter insertion or removal is within 8–12 h of the administration of LMWH.
- Patients at very high risk of VTE should be considered preoperatively for a temporary vena caval filter.
- Some national guidelines recommend 4 weeks of anti-coagulation after colonic and pelvic surgery, which currently can only be given by daily LMWH subcutaneous injection. Rivaroxaban, a direct inhibitor of activated factor X, has been introduced in orthopaedic surgery for prophylaxis of VTE after major joint replacement. It is yet to be studied in general surgical patients but has the advantage that it is in a simple once-daily tablet form.

Reducing the Risk of Wound Infection

- Prophylactic antibiotics should be administered as per local guidelines.
- Patients should be kept warm throughout the peri-operative period.
- Individualised goal-directed fluid therapy to optimise oxygen delivery to the tissues.

References

1. Boersma E, Kertai MD, Schouten O, Bax JJ, Noordzij P, Steyerberg EW, Schinkel AF, van Santen M, Simoons ML, Thomson IR, Klein J, van Urk H, Poldermans D. Perioperative cardiovascular mortality in noncardiac surgery: validation of the Lee cardiac risk index. Am J Med 2005;118:1134–1141.
2. Morris CK, Ueshima K, Kawaguchi T, Hideg A, Froelicher VF. The prognostic value of exercise capacity: a review of the literature. Am Heart J. 1991;122(5):1423–31.
3. Older P, Hall A, Hader R. Cardiopulmonary exercise testing as a screening test for perioperative management of major surgery in the elderly. Chest. 1999;116(2):355–62.
4. Older P, Smith R, Hall A, French C. Preoperative cardiopulmonary risk assessment by cardiopulmonary exercise testing. Crit Care Resusc. 2000;2(3):198–208.
5. Snowden CP, Prentis JM, Anderson HL, Roberts DR, Randles D, Renton M, et al. Submaximal cardiopulmonary exercise testing predicts complications and hospital length of stay in patients undergoing major elective surgery. Ann Surg. 2010;251(3):535–41.

6. Fleisher LA, Beckman JA, Brown KA, Calkins H, Chaikof E, Fleischmann KE, et al. ACC/AHA 2007 Guidelines on Perioperative Cardiovascular Evaluation and Care for Noncardiac Surgery: Executive Summary: A Report of the American College of Cardiology/American Heart Association Task Force on Practice Guidelines (Writing Committee to Revise the 2002 Guidelines on Perioperative Cardiovascular Evaluation for Noncardiac Surgery): Developed in Collaboration With the American Society of Echocardiography, American Society of Nuclear Cardiology, Heart Rhythm Society, Society of Cardiovascular Anesthesiologists, Society for Cardiovascular Angiography and Interventions, Society for Vascular Medicine and Biology, and Society for Vascular Surgery. Circulation. 2007;116(17):1971–96.

7. Levy BF, Scott MJ, Fawcett WJ, Rockall TA. 23-hour-stay laparoscopic colectomy. Dis Colon Rectum. 2009;52(7):1239–43.

8. Song F, Glenny AM. Antimicrobial prophylaxis in colorectal surgery: a systematic review of randomized controlled trials. Br J Surg. 1998;85(9):1232–41.

9. Basse L, Madsen JL, Kehlet H. Normal gastrointestinal transit after colonic resection using epidural analgesia, enforced oral nutrition and laxative. Br J Surg. 2001;88(11):1498–500.

10. McPhail MJ, Abu-Hilal M, Johnson CD. A meta-analysis comparing suprapubic and transurethral catheterization for bladder drainage after abdominal surgery. Br J Surg. 2006;93(9):1038–44.

11. Wong PF, Kumar S, Bohra A, Whetter D, Leaper DJ. Randomized clinical trial of perioperative systemic warming in major elective abdominal surgery. Br J Surg. 2007;94(4):421–6.

12. Kurz A, Sessler DI, Lenhardt R. Perioperative normothermia to reduce the incidence of surgical-wound infection and shorten hospitalization. Study of Wound Infection and Temperature Group. N Engl J Med. 1996;334(19):1209–15.

13. Scott EM, Buckland R. A systematic review of intraoperative warming to prevent postoperative complications. AORN J. 2006;83(5):1090–104, 1107–1013.

14. Frank SM, Fleisher LA, Breslow MJ, Higgins MS, Olson KF, Kelly S, et al. Perioperative maintenance of normothermia reduces the incidence of morbid cardiac events. A randomized clinical trial. JAMA. 1997;277(14):1127–34.

15. Apfel CC, Kranke P, Eberhart LH, Roos A, Roewer N. Comparison of predictive models for postoperative nausea and vomiting. Br J Anaesth. 2002;88(2):234–40.

16. Carlisle JB, Stevenson CA. Drugs for preventing postoperative nausea and vomiting. Cochrane Database Syst Rev 2006;(3):CD004125.

17. Mythen MG, Webb AR. Perioperative plasma volume expansion reduces the incidence of gut mucosal hypoperfusion during cardiac surgery. Arch Surg. 1995;130(4):423–9.

18. Gan TJ, Soppitt A, Maroof M, Ael-Moalem H, Robertson KM, Moretti E, et al. Goal-directed intraoperative fluid administration reduces length of hospital stay after major surgery. Anesthesiology. 2002;97(4):820–6.

19. Wakeling HG, McFall MR, Jenkins CS, Woods WG, Miles WF, Barclay GR, et al. Intraoperative oesophageal Doppler guided fluid management shortens postoperative hospital stay after major bowel surgery. Br J Anaesth. 2005;95(5):634–42.

20. Noblett SE, Snowden CP, Shenton BK, Horgan AF. Randomized clinical trial assessing the effect of Doppler-optimized fluid management on outcome after elective colorectal resection. Br J Surg. 2006;93(9):1069–76.

21. Conway DH, Mayall R, Abdul-Latif MS, Gilligan S, Tackaberry C. Randomised controlled trial investigating the influence of intravenous fluid titration using oesophageal Doppler monitoring during bowel surgery. Anaesthesia. 2002;57(9):845–9.

22. Hofer CK, Zalunardo MP, Klaghofer R, Spahr T, Pasch T, Zollinger A. Changes in intrathoracic blood volume associated with pneumoperitoneum and positioning. Acta Anaesthesiol Scand. 2002;46(3):303–8.

23. Falabella A, Moore-Jeffries E, Sullivan MJ, Nelson R, Lew M. Cardiac function during steep Trendelenburg position and CO2 pneumoperitoneum for robotic-assisted prostatectomy: a trans-oesophageal Doppler probe study. Int J Med Robot. 2007;3(4):312–5.

24. Rist M, Hemmerling TM, Rauh R, Siebzehnrubl E, Jacobi KE. Influence of pneumoperitoneum and patient positioning on preload and splanchnic blood volume in laparoscopic surgery of the lower abdomen. J Clin Anesth. 2001;13(4):244–9.

25. Levy B, Dowson H, Fawcett WJ, Scott MJP, Stoneham JR, Zuleika M, et al. The effect of regional anaesthesia on haemodynamic changes occurring during laparoscopic colorectal surgery. Anaesthesia. 2009;64(7):810.
26. Galizia G, Prizio G, Lieto E, Castellano P, Pelosio L, Imperatore V, et al. Hemodynamic and pulmonary changes during open, carbon dioxide pneumoperitoneum and abdominal wall-lifting cholecystectomy. A prospective, randomized study. Surg Endosc. 2001;15(5):477–83.
27. Alfonsi P, Vieillard-Baron A, Coggia M, Guignard B, Goeau-Brissonniere O, Jardin F, et al. Cardiac function during intraperitoneal CO2 insufflation for aortic surgery: a transesophageal echocardiographic study. Anesth Analg. 2006;102(5):1304–10.
28. Demyttenaere S, Feldman LS, Fried GM. Effect of pneumoperitoneum on renal perfusion and function: a systematic review. Surg Endosc. 2007;21(2):152–60.
29. Park EY, Koo BN, Min KT, Nam SH. The effect of pneumoperitoneum in the steep Trendelenburg position on cerebral oxygenation. Acta Anaesthesiol Scand. 2009;53(7): 895–9.
30. Levy B, Dowson H, Scott M, Stoneham J, Fawcett W, Zuleika M, et al. The effect of analgesic regime on post-operative lung function following laparoscopic colorectal surgery. BJS. 2008;95(S3):57.
31. Geerts WH, Heit JA, Clagett GP, Pineo GF, Colwell CW, Anderson Jr FA, et al. Prevention of venous thromboembolism. Chest. 2001;119(1 Suppl):132S–75.
32. Wille-Jorgensen P, Rasmussen MS, Andersen BR, Borly L. Heparins and mechanical methods for thromboprophylaxis in colorectal surgery. Cochrane Database Syst Rev 2001;(3): CD001217
33. Collins R, Scrimgeour A, Yusuf S, Peto R. Reduction in fatal pulmonary embolism and venous thrombosis by perioperative administration of subcutaneous heparin. Overview of results of randomized trials in general, orthopedic, and urologic surgery. N Engl J Med. 1988;318(18): 1162–73.
34. McLeod RS, Geerts WH, Sniderman KW, Greenwood C, Gregoire RC, Taylor BM, et al. Subcutaneous heparin versus low-molecular-weight heparin as thromboprophylaxis in patients undergoing colorectal surgery: results of the canadian colorectal DVT prophylaxis trial: a randomized, double-blind trial. Ann Surg. 2001;233(3):438–44.

Chapter 5
Perioperative Fluid Management in Enhanced Recovery

Krishna K. Varadhan and Dileep N. Lobo

Introduction

Intravenous fluid therapy is an integral component of perioperative care, but this has, till recently, often been based on little evidence and much dogma, and patients have received either too much or too little fluid. Unfortunately, the morbidity resultant from sub-optimal fluid therapy has often been lost in the seriousness of the conditions (such as sepsis and major trauma) that call for the use of fluids [1]. However, resurgence of interest in perioperative fluid therapy in the twenty-first century has yielded good evidence that optimal fluid management is an important determinant of surgical outcome and that, as far as possible, patients should be managed in a state of zero fluid balance, avoiding both overload and underhydration [2–5].

Surgical dogma has often led to prolonged periods of preoperative starvation [6], which, apart from inducing insulin resistance, also causes patients to reach the anaesthetic room in a state of fluid depletion [7], which may be further compounded by indiscriminate bowel preparation [8], another practice that has not been shown to have a positive effect on surgical outcome [9]. On the other hand, the concept that patients should receive large amounts of salt-containing fluids in the perioperative period leads to a state of salt and water overload that can also affect surgical outcomes adversely [5, 10–17].

K.K. Varadhan
Division of Gastrointestinal Surgery, Nottingham Digestive
Diseases Centre NIHR Biomedical Research Unit,
Nottingham University Hospitals, Queen's Medical Centre,
Nottingham, Notts, UK

D.N. Lobo (✉)
Nottingham Digestive Diseases Centre NIHR Biomedical Research Unit,
Nottingham University Hospitals, Queen's Medical Centre,
Nottingham, Notts, UK

N. Francis et al. (eds.), *Manual of Fast Track Recovery for Colorectal Surgery*,
Enhanced Recovery, DOI 10.1007/978-0-85729-953-6_5,
© Springer-Verlag London Limited 2012

The Enhanced Recovery After Surgery (ERAS) protocol [18] has recognised the importance of optimisation of fluid delivery and avoidance of fluid overload in managing patients in a state of metabolic equilibrium and improving outcomes, the evidence base for which is discussed in this chapter.

Pathophysiology of Inappropriate Fluid Balance

The ultimate goal of perioperative intravenous fluid therapy is to maintain tissue perfusion and cellular oxygen delivery, while at the same time keeping the patient in a state of zero fluid balance if possible. However, prior to the warning on the adverse effects of excessive fluid administration issued by Moore and Shires [3], it was common surgical practice to replace blood loss with three times the volume of crystalloid and to provide extra fluid for so called 'third-space losses'. Although the daily maintenance requirements for sodium and water are estimated at 1 mmol/kg and 25–35 mL/kg, respectively, to support the integrity of the extracellular fluid volume, it has not been unusual for patients to receive in excess of 5 L water and 700 mmol sodium/day in the early postoperative period [10, 12, 13, 16, 19, 20]. In evolutionary terms, the well-developed metabolic response to trauma is to conserve salt and water in order to preserve intravascular volume. However, when excess fluid is administered, most of the excess accumulates in the extravascular compartment and causes oedema [21], which is detrimental to surgical outcome [11, 12, 22].

'Normal' saline or 0.9% sodium chloride is one of the most frequently used intravenous crystalloids in general surgical practice and ten million litres of this solution are used in the UK each year. A survey published in 2001 suggested that over a quarter of junior doctors in the UK were prescribing ≥2 L of 0.9% saline per day to meet what they supposed to be maintenance requirements in the postoperative period [19], although this volume provides more than four times the normal daily requirement of sodium and chloride, and results inevitably in salt and water overload with all its problems. An examination of the history of 0.9% saline reveals very little scientific basis for its use [23], which is mostly based on custom and convenience. The origins of 0.9% saline supposedly date from the salt solutions pioneered during the 1831–1832 cholera epidemic that swept across north-east England, although the solutions used at that time were, in fact, quite different with much lower salt concentrations [23]. The use of 0.9% saline originated from the in vitro studies of Hartold Jacob Hamburger who, in the 1890s, found that the freezing point of 0.9% saline was the same as that of human serum (i.e. iso-osmolar) and that erythrocytes were least likely to undergo lysis in this solution [23–25]. Hamburger called this solution 'indifferent' saline, indicating that it had no effect on the red blood cells. Somehow, this term got corrupted to 'physiological' or 'normal' [23]. It is uncertain when 0.9% saline was first used intravenously in human patients, but the side effects of administering large amounts of 0.9% saline soon became apparent [1].

While there is no doubt that 0.9% sodium chloride has saved many lives, this has probably been achieved at the expense of avoidable morbidity. The solution is far from physiological [23, 26, 27]; its content of sodium, 154 mmol/L, being nearly 10% higher, and of chloride, 154 mmol/L, 50% higher than that in extracellular fluid. A review of the literature fails to reveal a single study showing it to be superior to more physiological crystalloids for resuscitation, replacement or maintenance. There are two randomised clinical trials in humans comparing 0.9% saline with Ringer's lactate in the perioperative period, showing that 0.9% saline caused more side effects [28, 29]. One of these studies, involving patients undergoing renal transplantation, had to be stopped prematurely because, compared with none in those receiving Ringer's lactate, 19% of patients in the saline group had to be treated for hyperkalaemia and 31% for metabolic acidosis [9]. In the other study, involving patients undergoing abdominal aortic aneurysm repair, those receiving saline needed more blood products and bicarbonate therapy [29]. A comprehensive review of the use of 0.9% saline for resuscitation has recommended that its routine use in massive fluid resuscitation should be discouraged [30].

Teleologically, mammals have developed very efficient mechanisms to conserve salt and water in the face of fluctuations in water supply and scarcity of salt. On the other hand we have not, until recent times, been exposed to salt excess and our mechanism for excreting this is correspondingly inefficient, depending on a slow and sustained suppression of the renin-angiotensin-aldosterone axis [21, 31]. Atrial natriuretic peptide seems to be more responsive to changes in intravascular volume than to total extracellular salt content. Even healthy human volunteers can take over 2 days to excrete a rapid infusion of 2 L of 0.9% saline [21, 31]. Most of the retained fluid after such infusions accumulates in the interstitial compartment [21, 31], leading to manifest oedema if overload exceeds 2–3 L [32, 33]. In the face of acute illness, injury or surgery, and also of severe malnutrition, the capacity to excrete a salt and water load is further impaired, only returning to normal during convalescence [34, 35]. An overload of 0.9% saline in such cases can cause hyperosmolar states [36], hyperchloraemic acidosis [21, 31–33, 37, 38], decreased renal blood flow and glomerular filtration rate [39], which in turn exacerbates sodium retention. Oedema impairs pulmonary gas exchange and tissue oxygenation, and leads to an increase in tissue pressure in organs such as the kidney, which are surrounded by a non-expansible capsule, thereby compromising microvascular perfusion, increasing arterio-venous shunting and reducing lymphatic drainage, all of which facilitate further oedema formation. Fluid accumulation in the lungs also increases the risk of pneumonia. Removal of excess alveolar fluid is achieved by active sodium transport and the gradient between the hydrostatic and colloid osmotic pressures. Active sodium transport is affected by fluid administration and by the release of pro-inflammatory cytokines, both of which occur perioperatively [40]. Acidosis impairs cardiac contractility, reduces responsiveness to inotropes, decreases renal perfusion and can be lethal in combination with hypothermia and coagulopathy [30]. Hyperchloraemic acidosis, as a result of saline infusions [21, 32, 33, 38, 41], has been shown to reduce gastric blood flow and decrease gastric intramucosal pH in elderly surgical patients [37], and both respiratory and metabolic acidosis have been associated with impaired gastric motility [13, 42, 43]. Just as fluid overload causes peripheral oedema, it may also cause splanchnic oedema resulting in increased abdominal pressure, ascites [44] and even the abdominal compartment syndrome [45]. Consequently, this may lead to a decrease in mesenteric blood flow and a further exacerbation of the process, leading to ileus or functional obstruction of anastomoses, increased gut permeability, intestinal failure and even anastomotic

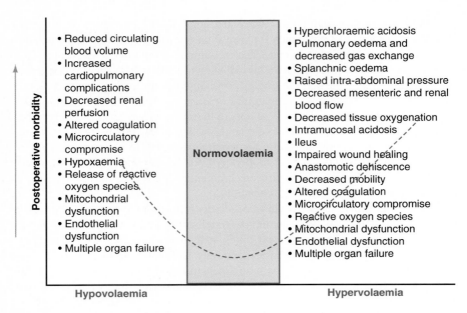

Fig. 5.1 The range for safe fluid therapy (Adapted from Bellamy [52])

dehiscence [11, 12, 14, 46, 47]. Fluid excess may also impair postoperative mobility and increase the risk of deep vein thrombosis [47], nausea, vomiting, abdominal pain, hyperventilation, headaches, thirst, confusion and diplopia [38].

At the cellular level saline excess can cause cytosolic acidification, membrane hyperpolarisation, inactivation of protein kinases, disruption of phosphorylation, impairment of mitochondrial function, inflammation, disordered neurotransmitter metabolism and poor glycaemic control [48]. Both Sydney Ringer [49] and Harvey Cushing [50] have shown that muscle contractility ceases in vitro when tissues are bathed in 0.9% saline.

On the other hand, true fluid restriction resulting in underhydration can be equally detrimental [51, 52] by resulting in decreased venous return and cardiac output, diminished tissue perfusion and oxygen delivery, increased blood viscosity, decreased saliva production with a predisposition to postoperative parotitis, and an increase in viscosity of pulmonary mucus resulting in mucous plug formation and ateletactasis [53]. Induction of anaesthesia in patients with a fluid deficit further reduces the effective circulatory volume by decreasing sympathetic tone. Inadequate fluid resuscitation and decreased tissue perfusion can lead to gastrointestinal mucosal acidosis and poorer outcome [54] (Fig. 5.1).

Compared with 0.9% saline, the use of balanced salt solutions, e.g. Hartmann's or Ringer's lactate/acetate, achieves better acid–base balance, less blood loss, better renal function, less nausea and vomiting, and probably better survival. In 1986 Veech wrote, 'The use of 0.9% saline imposes unnecessary demands of a widespread nature upon cellular energy metabolism until the kidney can excrete the excessive chloride infused. This is unnecessary today in light of the technical advances in the last 50 years' [26].

Types of Fluids

Salt (sodium chloride) containing crystalloids and colloids are used during resuscitation to expand the intravascular volume. The ability of a solution to expand the plasma volume is dependent on its volume of distribution and the metabolic fate of the solute, so that while colloids are mainly distributed in the intravascular compartment, once the dextrose is metabolised, dextrose-containing solutions are distributed through the total body water and, hence, have a limited and transient capacity to expand blood volume. Isotonic sodium-containing crystalloids are distributed throughout the extracellular volume, including the plasma, and textbook teaching classically suggests that such infusions expand the blood volume by one-third the volume of crystalloid infused [55]. In practice, however, the efficiency of these solutions to expand the plasma volume is only between 20% and 25%, the remainder being sequestered in the interstitial space [21, 56, 57]. Although these solutions are used successfully for this purpose, the price paid for adequate intravascular filling is overexpansion of the interstitial space and tissue oedema. Solutions of dextrose or of hypotonic saline can cause significant hyponatraemia ($Na^+ < 130$ mmol/L) when used in excess, and care should be taken to avoid this potentially harmful effect, particularly in children and the elderly [58].

Colloids are fluids that contain particles large enough to be retained within the circulation and, therefore, to exert an oncotic pressure across the capillary membrane. Albumin solutions are monodisperse as they contain particles of uniform molecular weight while synthetic colloids contain particles of varying sizes and molecular weights in an attempt to optimise the half-life and plasma volume-expanding capacities of the solutions [59, 60]. Colloids are more efficient at staying in the intravascular space and in producing less interstitial oedema than crystalloids. The blood volume expanding effect of colloids such as hydroxyethyl starch is in the range of 60–70% [21, 31]. Colloids may also improve microcirculatory flow [61] and are more anti- than pro-coagulant. However, the evidence from systematic reviews and meta-analyses does not show that resuscitation with colloids confers an advantage in reducing the risk of death compared to crystalloids in patients with trauma, burns and following surgery or that one colloid is more effective than others [62–65]. Moreover, crystalloids have found to be much more cost-effective for fluid optimization [66, 67].

Fluid Therapy in Colorectal Surgery

Surgery for colorectal cancer is associated with an overall mortality risk of <5%, with 70% of patients being over the age of 65 years [68] with poor functional reserve and associated co-morbidities. The internal milieu of patients undergoing colorectal surgery is subjected to physiological alterations in the composition of water and electrolytes in the various fluid compartments as determined by the nature of disease process, type of surgery, anaesthesia, acute blood loss and the perioperative care [69].

Restrictive/Standard/Liberal Regimens

Several studies have examined the effect of different fluid regimens on postoperative outcomes following colorectal surgery. Whilst showing good postoperative outcomes for individual regimens, there were no clear definitions or standardisation for volume and type of fluids, making direct comparisons and interpretation of these studies difficult. Some studies have suggested that 'restrictive' fluid therapy is associated with good outcome in patients having major abdominal surgery [10, 13, 70, 71], while others have suggested that 'restricted' fluid regimens may be detrimental to outcome [51, 72].

Lobo et al. [13] studied the effect of salt and water balance on recovery of gastrointestinal function after elective colonic resection and set the tone for a radical change in the perioperative fluid management of surgical patients and evoked interest for further studies in this area. The standard group received a minimum of 3 L of intravenous fluid with 154 mmol of sodium each day, while the restricted group received no more than 2 L water with 77 mmol of sodium. Apart from resulting in positive salt and water balance with a 3 kg gain in weight, the standard regimen resulted in a delay in recovery of gastric emptying and prolonged hospital stay. Moreover, despite fluid restriction to 2 L, none of the patients in the restricted group developed renal impairment or hyponatraemia. This was the first study to demonstrate that fluid overload could result in gastrointestinal failure.

These results were supported by those of Brandstrup et al. [10] who randomised 141 patients undergoing elective colorectal resection to standard or restricted intra- and postoperative fluid management in an observer-blinded multi-centre trial. The patients in the restricted group were not given intravenous fluids for pre-loading or replacement for third-space losses and were encouraged to have oral fluids postoperatively. The regimens used were complex, but in simplistic terms, the standard group were given fluids to increase body weight while in hospital by 3–7 kg, while those in the restricted group were maintained in a state of zero fluid balance. The fluid-restricted group had an earlier return of bowel function and 50% fewer complications, compared to the standard group. Interestingly, the authors also reported a dose–response relation between complications and increasing volumes of intravenous fluid ($p < 0.001$) as well as increasing body weight ($p < 0.001$) on the day of operation, independent of allocation group. There were four deaths in the standard group due to cardiorespiratory complications and none were reported in the fluid-restricted group.

Two other studies reported the effects of 'standard' versus 'restrictive' fluid regimes, in patients undergoing vascular surgery. McArdle et al. [16] compared the effects the two regimens during both intra- and postoperative periods, in patients undergoing open elective infra-renal abdominal aortic aneurysm repair while Gonzalez-Fajardo et al. [73] studied the effect of 'restrictive' fluid therapy with a 'standard' regime, postoperatively. Both these studies reported significantly increased risk of complications and length of stay in the 'standard' group, compared with the 'fluid-restricted' group. The cumulative fluid balance was also similarly 'less positive' in the restricted groups in both studies.

Holte et al. [72] randomised 32 consecutive patients undergoing elective colonic surgery to 'restrictive' and 'liberal' fluid regimen using Ringer's lactate during the intraoperative period. The pre- and postoperative fluid management were standardised according to protocol. They failed to show any significant differences in terms of intraoperative haemodynamic parameters or cardiorespiratory function. No significant differences were reported in the number of re-admissions or complications rates. However, there was a trend (statistically not significant) towards increased risk of anastomotic leakage in the restrictive group.

These results were similar to the study by McKay et al. [74], in which 80 patients were randomised to receive either a restricted regimen of less than 2 L of water and 77 mmol sodium for 24 h after surgery or a standard regimen of 3 L water and 154 mmol sodium per day for 3 days postoperatively. There were no significant differences on postoperative gastrointestinal function, complications, hospital stay or mortality. These results were attributed to a conservative approach to intraoperative fluid and sodium management, avoiding gross fluid gains, resulting in minimal differences in the total fluid given and a change of median bodyweight within 1 kg of preoperative values in both groups.

In contrast, the study by Nisanevich et al. [15] evaluated the effects of 'liberal' and 'restrictive' fluid regimens using lactated Ringer's solution in the intraoperative period. Although there were significant differences in the amount of fluids administered intraoperatively (3.8 vs. 1.4 L), the amounts given postoperatively were similar. Interestingly, they reported significantly better outcomes in the fluid restricted group with regards to complications, return of bowel function, weight gain and hospital stay.

An attempt to study the risk of surgical wound infection following colonic surgery was made by Kabon et al. [75], by the use of supplemental Ringer's solution, comparing 'small' with 'large' fluid management during surgery. This resulted in large-volume patients receiving almost twice as much total fluid compared to small-volume patients (5.7 ± 2 vs. 3.1 ± 1.5 L). However, the results failed to show any significant differences in wound infections, bowel function or duration of hospitalisation.

A recent study by Vermeulen et al. [51] compared standard versus restrictive fluid therapy after major abdominal surgery. Duration and type of surgical procedures were similar in both groups. No significant differences were found between both groups for any of the gastrointestinal function parameters, time to removal of nasogastric tubes and discontinuation of intravenous and epidural catheters. Neither group was maintained in a state of fluid balance, but there were more complications and protocol violations in the restricted group.

An attempt to clarify the terms 'restrictive', 'standard' and 'liberal' using the total amount of fluids given in the control and intervention arms of randomised controlled studies was made in a meta-analysis performed by us [5], in which the groups were standardised as follows: restricted fluid therapy: <1.75 L/day; liberal fluid therapy/ fluid overload: >2.75 L/day; fluid balance: between 1.75 and 2.75 L/day.

Based on these definitions, patients who received more or less fluid than those who received a balanced amount were considered to be in a state of 'fluid imbalance'. Nine studies [10, 13, 15, 16, 51, 72–75] with a total of 801 patients met the inclusion criteria for the meta-analysis. Using the original definitions as described in the individual studies, 'restricted' fluid regimens when compared with 'standard or liberal' fluid regimens, showed no difference in postoperative complication rates (risk ratio 0.83 (95% CI 0.49, 1.39, $p=0.47$)) or length of hospital stay (weighted mean difference (WMD) -1.77 (95% CI -4.36, 0.81) d, $p=0.18$).

However, applying standardised definitions (balance vs. imbalance), the results showed there was a 59% reduction in risk of developing complications in the group that was in a state of fluid balance when compared with the group in imbalance and there was a 3.4-day reduction in hospital stay in the former group. When studies using primarily 0.9% saline were analysed, similar results were observed with a 49% reduction in complications and a 4.4-day reduction in length of hospital stay [5]. Moreover, maximum weight gain was seen in the studies in which the standard group received an excessive amount of fluid [10, 13, 15]. It appears that patients need to gain at least 2.5–3 kg in weight, as a result of salt and water overload, in the postoperative period in order to have a worse outcome than those maintained in a state of zero fluid balance [76]. Avoidance of fluid overload, rather than fluid restriction, seems to be the key to better postoperative outcome [12].

Cardiovascular Monitoring

Conventional intraoperative monitoring techniques may not predict accurate fluid requirements since they are based on mean arterial pressure (MAP), which is dependent on both cardiac output (CO) and systemic vascular resistance (SVR) and, thus not a good indicator of blood flow or oxygen delivery [77]. Optimal fluid therapy requires clear preoperative decision making to monitor haemodynamic stability during the perioperative period, usually determined from information based on a thorough clinical assessment taking into account the co-morbidities, nature of disease process, surgery, anticipated blood loss and the level of care needed postoperatively. In addition to helping optimise cardiac output and oxygen delivery, cardiovascular monitoring also assists in differentiating between varying aetiologies of haemodynamic instability including hypovolaemia, sepsis and cardiogenic causes of tissue hypoperfusion or shock [78].

Haemodynamic variables such as mean arterial pressure and cardiac output are directly related to the heart rate and stroke volume. Whilst invasive monitoring methods such as measurement of venous (CVP) pressure using a cannula and a pressure transducer gives an indication of the preload, arterial cannulation gives a beat-to-beat arterial pressure waveform, which helps assess myocardial performance, preload and systemic vascular resistance. However, it must be noted that these measurements must be interpreted with the knowledge of the patients' past medical history and current physiology. Moreover, measurement of cardiac output and stroke volume itself does not directly reflect oxygen delivery (DO_2), since overzealous fluid administration using a pre-determined regimen and end point can restore cardiac output at the expense of reduced oxygen carrying capacity and thus DO_2 (normal: 600 mL/m²). To offset this problem, the estimation of beat-to-beat Hb and SpO_2 (Masimo Radical 7, Masimo Corporation, California, USA), if used alongside continuous measurement of CO, will allow real time assessment of DO_2 [79].

Intraoperative transoesophageal Doppler (TOD) probes for continuous monitoring of cardiac output enable optimisation of intravascular volume and tissue perfusion in major abdominal surgery. They are associated with a reduction in the incidence of postoperative complications and length of hospital stay and can be very useful in high-risk patients. The TOD monitor is a relatively non-invasive method of measuring cardiac output using a flexible 4 MHz ultrasound probe placed in the oesophagus to insonate the descending aorta and the Doppler principle to measure peak blood flow velocity and the flow time, which is corrected for the heart rate. Pearse and colleagues [80], in their study using the LiDCO system, a minimally invasive indicator (lithium) dilution technique, and pulse contour power analysis of radial artery waveform to measure stroke volume and thus cardiac output, concluded that goal-directed therapy reduces hospital stay, postoperative nausea and vomiting and complications, and facilitates faster gastrointestinal functional recovery. Similar favourable results have reported by others using LiDCO [81–83], although within the criteria specified for such monitors, the limited ability of LiDCO to track rapid changes in SV as a result of major haemorrhage in animal models or use of vasoactive agents have been highlighted. However other non-invasive flow-related techniques to optimise intraoperative fluid therapy have shown varied results compared to the oesophageal Doppler guided-GDT [82, 84, 85]. But, to realize the full benefit of such high-level monitoring devices, fluid optimisation should extend into the postoperative period.

Goal-Directed Therapy

Intraoperative fluid therapy guided by evidence-based protocols and advances in flow monitors with the understanding of fluid pathophysiology have had a positive influence on enhanced recovery outcomes. The principles of goal-directed therapy (GDT) are based on measurements of cardiac output or other similar parameters to guide intravenous fluid and inotropic therapy. Many studies using GDT have reported improved short-term outcomes in patients undergoing major abdominal surgery [86–89]. GDT is also supported by the British Consensus Guidelines on Intravenous Therapy for Adult Surgical Patients (GIFTASUP) [4] published in 2008, which state, 'In patients undergoing abdominal surgery, intraoperative treatment with intravenous fluid to achieve an optimal value of stroke volume should be used where possible as this may reduce postoperative complication rates and duration of hospital stay. Level 1a'.

A number of clinical studies have reported that administering fluids to achieve maximal left ventricular stroke volume whilst avoiding excess fluid administration and consequent impairment of left ventricular performance improves outcomes in patients undergoing major general surgery, especially when commenced preoperatively [80, 90–93]. It is to be noted that a majority of patients presented with a functional preoperative volume deficit and in a fraction of these patients, the deficit was of clinical relevance needing optimisation by maximising stroke volume with a median of 200 mL, emphasising the need for an individualised approach to GDT [94].

Two meta-analyses [2, 95] that compared goal directed with conventional therapy in patients having abdominal surgery reported a reduced incidence of postoperative complications and length of stay. Walsh et al. [95] reported that paradoxically, there was no difference in the amount of intraoperative crystalloid and colloid administered between the groups and concluded that this might be due to high heterogeneity in the analysis of colloid volumes and, hence, the data should be interpreted with caution. On the contrary, other studies reported using significantly more colloid in the Doppler-guided group [86, 88, 89].

In the study by Wakeling et al. [89], intraoperative oesophageal Doppler-guided fluid management was associated with a 1.5-day median reduction in postoperative hospital stay and 22% reduction in complications. Patients recovered gut function significantly faster and suffered significantly less gastrointestinal and overall morbidity [89]. This was similar to the study by Noblett et al. [86], which showed that the use of oesophageal Doppler and LiDCO cardiac monitors was associated with a reduction in morbidity and length of stay after major surgery.

The use of Doppler-guided fluid therapy has been shown to reduce the complications and length of stay in other specialities, including hip surgery [96, 97] and urology/gynaecology [88]. Measures to improve oxygen delivery using inotropes have been reported to improve outcomes after major elective surgery with significant reduction in mortality and morbidity in high-risk surgical patients [91, 93]. However, the study by Stone et al. [98], giving fluid infusions during surgery using stroke volume measurements guided by oesophageal Doppler to increase cardiac output, failed to show a significant difference between inotrope use and saline, in terms of postoperative complications or length of stay and suggested that fluid optimisation is the major contributor to improved oxygen delivery. Davies et al. [99] also did not show any significant advantages of dopexamine use in high-risk patients receiving goal-directed fluid therapy undergoing major abdominal surgery.

Similarly, the importance of fluid optimisation using GDT over inotrope use is supported by a systematic review [2], which reported reduced hospital stay, fewer complications and intensive care unit (ICU) admissions, less requirement for inotropes and early return of gastrointestinal function in the group managed by GDT. Despite these clinical and economic advantages, the use of GDT or other minimally invasive techniques have not been adopted widely or become universally available in the operating theatres [52].

Fluid Therapy Within an ERAS Protocol

The important concepts of the ERAS protocol are based on best evidence that enables an accelerated recovery from surgery with the aim of minimising the stress response, thereby reducing morbidity and mortality [18]. In contrast to traditional care methods, ERAS uses a structured care pathway. The main components affecting perioperative fluid balance are summarised in Table 5.1.

Preoperative

No Pre-medication

The role of anaesthetists is critical in successful delivery of fast-track surgery programs [100]. One of the aims of the preoperative assessment should be that patients should reach anaesthetic room in a state of adequate hydration [76]. The importance of appropriate use of anaesthetic agents, inotropes and prophylactic drugs to minimise side effects, fluids and blood transfusions in the perioperative period cannot be overemphasised.

Preoperative assessment of fluid deficit in patients having major colorectal surgery should include a clear history of presenting illness with regards to the duration of gastrointestinal symptoms such as vomiting or diarrhoea, decreased oral intake, length of preoperative fasting, preoperative bowel preparation and evidence of dehydration on physical examination. These should be corroborated with laboratory values of haemoglobin, urea, nitrogen and creatinine, as clinical examination alone may not predict accurate fluid deficit [101, 102]. Long-acting sedatives, hypnotics and opioids are associated with prolonged recovery due to inability to drink or mobilise postoperatively. Therefore, short-acting medications are recommended to facilitate early recovery.

Mechanical Bowel Preparation

Routine mechanical bowel preparation contribute to preoperative fluid deficit, especially in the elderly [103]. Reports from studies suggest no benefit, [104] or rather an increased risk of complications such as prolonged postoperative ileus as well as increased risk of anastomotic leakage from mechanical bowel preparation [9, 105–108]. Some studies indicated that a calculated volume of intravenous fluid administered during bowel preparation improves patient outcomes with respect to blood transfusion and postoperative oliguria [8, 109]. However, it has been reported that with hypertonic bowel preparations (e.g. sodium phosphate), increased plasma osmalility, urea and phosphate concentrations, decreased calcium and potassium can result even in healthy volunteers [103]. Therefore the consensus guidelines from the

Table 5.1 Recommendations for fluid therapy for patients managed under an ERAS protocol

Preoperative
- Preoperative starvation leads to fluid depletion – solid food intake should be allowed up to 6 h and clear liquids (including carbohydrate loading) up to 2 h before induction of anaesthesia.
- Mechanical bowel preparation leads to loss of salt and water. If bowel preparation is necessary, patients should be rehydrated to their pre-bowel preparation body weight prior to arrival in the anaesthetic room.

Intraoperative
- Colloid boluses to optimize cardiac output, as measured by transoesophageal Doppler, lead to less interstitial overload and better outcomes. Other monitoring devices such as LiDCO may be used.
- Intraoperative crystalloid overload should be avoided, especially with unbalanced solutions such as 0.9% saline.
- Balanced crystalloids and colloids are preferable to 0.9% saline-based fluids.
- Significant blood loss should be replaced by 1:1:1 transfusions of packed cells, fresh frozen plasma and platelets.
- Intraoperative hypotension in the euvolaemic patient may be controlled with vasopressors.

Postoperative
- Avoidance of nasogastric tubes and prevention and treatment of postoperative nausea and vomiting leads to better oral fluid and nutrient intake and reduces the need for intravenous fluid.
- The euvolaemic patient requires no more than 2–2.5 L water and 70–100 mmol sodium intravenously per day. Potassium supplements should be added. Most patients require intravenous fluids for no more than 48 h after colonic surgery.
- Epidural analgesia–induced hypotension in the adequately hydrated patient should be treated with vasopressors. If necessary a 250–500 mL bolus of balanced colloid rather than crystalloid should be used.
- As far as possible, patients should be managed in a state of zero fluid balance, avoiding both overhydration and underhydration. Overhydration leading to short-term weight gain >2.5 kg is detrimental to outcome.

ERAS society recommend that 'patients undergoing elective colonic resection above the peritoneal reflection should not receive routine oral bowel preparation. Bowel preparation may be considered in patients scheduled for low rectal resection where a diverting stoma is planned' [18].

Preoperative Fasting

ERAS principles emphasise avoidance of prolonged fasting as overnight preoperative fasting and metabolic stress from surgery leads to fluid deficits and postoperative insulin resistance [110]. It has been shown that the degree of insulin resistance is related to the magnitude of the operation [111]. Provision of food up to 6 h preoperatively and clear carbohydrate drinks up to 2 h preoperatively ensures that patients are in metabolically fed state, reduces preoperative thirst, anxiety, postoperative nausea and vomiting and also improves insulin sensitivity, even in diabetic patients [112]. Overnight fasting does not reduce the risk of aspiration and intake of clear fluids until 2 h before anaesthesia is as safe [113]. There is also evidence to suggest that shortened preoperative fasting does not increase the risk of aspiration, regurgitation or related morbidity compared with the standard 'nil by mouth from midnight' [113]. Thus, ERAS recommendations are that ' the duration of preoperative fasting should be 2 h for liquids and 6 h for solids and patients should receive carbohydrate loading preoperatively' [18].

Intraoperative

Fluid Optimisation

There is increasing evidence to suggest that excess salt and water is associated with inhibition of gastrointestinal function, pulmonary complications, immobility and prolonged recovery [13, 42, 47, 114–116]. A typical weight gain of 3–6 kg has been reported in colonic surgery [13, 117]. Many studies have reported that intravenous fluid therapy that does not change body weight reduces postoperative complications [10], reduces bowel wall oedema and preserves anastomotic stability [13, 14]. Weight gain in excess of 20% has been shown to be associated with increased morbidity among postoperative patients in intensive care [118].

Therefore, the aim of a GDT should be to optimise intravascular volume to ensure adequate tissue perfusion. Intraoperative optimisation of fluid therapy should aim to use intravenous fluids efficiently, relevant to the patient's needs. When possible, preload should be optimised before administering vasoactive drugs as any preoperative fluid and electrolyte derangements may exacerbate hypovolaemia and complicate intra- and postoperative fluid management. Monitoring of haemodynamic variables guided by GDT should be considered on an individual basis to aid fluid therapy in certain high-risk patients. This should be achieved by efficient use of fluids guided by the cardiovascular parameters and careful monitoring of the response throughout the perioperative period to maintain cardiac output and stroke volume.

Mid-thoracic Epidural Analgesia

Preoperative commencement of a mid-thoracic epidural blocks stress hormone release and attenuates postoperative insulin resistance [18]. It also helps in achieving analgesia and sympathetic blockade and in preventing gut paralysis [119]. ERAS programmes recommend continuous low-dose mid-thoracic epidural using local anaesthetic and opioid combinations for approximately 48 h, following elective colonic surgery and approximately 72–96 h after pelvic surgery with boluses for breakthrough pain. Paracetamol (acetaminophen) (4 g/d) for baseline analgesia and NSAIDs following removal of epidural should be started postoperatively.

Treatment of Postoperative Nausea and Vomiting (PONV)

Aggressive treatment of PONV facilitates early oral feeding. Symptoms related to postoperative ileus and opioids can be more stressful than postoperative pain. Female gender, non-smoking status, history of motion sickness or PONV and postoperative opioids confer high risk [120, 121]. Individuals at moderate risk (>2 factors) should receive prophylactically with dexamethosone sodium phosphate at induction or serotonin receptor antagonist at the end of surgery [122, 123].

Avoid Nasogastric Tubes

Avoiding routine use of nasogastric tubes is associated with earlier return of gastrointestinal function and is not associated with increased risk of anastomotic leak or length of stay [124]. Routine use of intra-abdominal drains in colonic or rectal surgery does not reduce the risk of complications. Drains should not be used for routine colonic resections above peritoneal reflections and for low anterior resections only short-term (<24 h) drainage should be considered.

Postoperative

Encourage Early Postoperative Oral Intake

Methods to establish early oral intake not only facilitates early return of bowel function, but also allows stopping of intravenous drips and aids mobilisation, leading to faster recovery. It reduces postoperative morbidity and is not associated with an increased risk of anastomotic dehiscence [125].

Avoid Fluid Overload

Avoidance of excessive hydration is essential whilst optimising maintenance requirements in the uncomplicated patient. Stopping intravenous fluids as early as possible and commencing oral fluids is the best available option to restrict fluid overload in the postoperative period. Most patients require no more than 2–2.5 L of water and 70–100 mmol of sodium per day. Potassium is best avoided on postoperative days 0 and 1, unless the serum potassium is low. However, regular potassium supplements should be prescribed from day 2 onwards.

The early postoperative phase is associated with oliguria, salt and water retention. Oliguria should be assessed as average urine output over 4 h and if associated with hypotension should be treated with fluid boluses of crystalloids or colloids titrated to patient response guided by flow-based therapy when possible, along with the correction of any fluid deficits, electrolyte abnormalities, careful monitoring of continuing losses and daily weighing. Hypovolaemia secondary to gastrointestinal losses from diarrhoea, ileus, small bowel fistula and ileostomy should be replaced volume for volume with balanced crystalloids. Blood transfusions if needed should be provided in the ratio of 1:1:1 of whole blood: FFP: platelets, as appropriate. However, oliguria, which is associated with epidural anaesthesia, is usually due to vasodilatation or relative intravascular hypovolaemia, and can be treated by judicious use of vasopressors [126].

Conclusion

Perioperative fluid therapy has a direct effect on outcome, and prescriptions should be tailored to the needs of the patient. The goal of fluid therapy in patients undergoing elective surgery is to maintain the effective circulatory volume while avoiding interstitial fluid overload whenever possible. Weight gain in elective surgical patients should be minimised in an attempt to achieve a 'zero fluid balance status'. On the other hand, patients should arrive in the anaesthetic room in a state of adequate hydration so as to avoid the need to resuscitate fluid-depleted patients in the anaesthetic room or after the induction of anaesthesia.

Optimal fluid delivery should be part of an overall care package that involves minimisation of the period of preoperative fasting, preoperative carbohydrate loading, thoracic epidural analgesia, avoidance of nasogastric tubes, early mobilisation and early return to oral feeding, as exemplified by the enhanced recovery after surgery programme [18]. There is a relatively narrow range for safe fluid therapy and too much or too little fluid can affect outcome adversely. Balance is the key [5].

References

1. Evans GH. The abuse of normal salt solution. JAMA. 1911;57:2126–7.
2. Abbas SM, Hill AG. Systematic review of the literature for the use of oesophageal Doppler monitor for fluid replacement in major abdominal surgery. Anaesthesia. 2008;63:44–51.
3. Moore FD, Shires G. Moderation. Ann Surg. 1967;166:300–1.
4. Powell-Tuck J, Gosling P, Lobo DN, Allison SP, Carlson GL, Gore M, et al. British consensus guidelines on intravenous fluid therapy for adult surgical patients. GIFTASUP. 2008. Available from: http://www.bapen.org.uk/pdfs/bapen_pubs/giftasup.pdf. Accessed 1 Jan 2011.
5. Varadhan KK, Lobo DN. A meta-analysis of randomised controlled trials of intravenous fluid therapy in major elective open abdominal surgery: getting the balance right. Proc Nutr Soc. 2010;69:488–98.
6. Maltby JR. Fasting from midnight–the history behind the dogma. Best Pract Res Clin Anaesthesiol. 2006;20:363–78.
7. Ljungqvist O, Soreide E. Preoperative fasting. Br J Surg. 2003;90:400–6.
8. Sanders G, Mercer SJ, Saeb-Parsey K, Akhavani MA, Hosie KB, Lambert AW. Randomized clinical trial of intravenous fluid replacement during bowel preparation for surgery. Br J Surg. 2001;88:1363–5.

9. Slim K, Vicaut E, Launay-Savary MV, Contant C, Chipponi J. Updated systematic review and meta-analysis of randomized clinical trials on the role of mechanical bowel preparation before colorectal surgery. Ann Surg. 2009;249:203–9.

10. Brandstrup B, Tonnesen H, Beier-Holgersen R, Hjortso E, Ording H, Lindorff-Larsen K, et al. Effects of intravenous fluid restriction on postoperative complications: comparison of two perioperative fluid regimens: a randomized assessor-blinded multicenter trial. Ann Surg. 2003;238:641–8.

11. Lobo DN. Sir David Cuthbertson medal lecture. Fluid, electrolytes and nutrition: physiological and clinical aspects. Proc Nutr Soc. 2004;63:453–66.

12. Lobo DN. Fluid overload and surgical outcome: another piece in the jigsaw. Ann Surg. 2009;249:186–8.

13. Lobo DN, Bostock KA, Neal KR, Perkins AC, Rowlands BJ, Allison SP. Effect of salt and water balance on recovery of gastrointestinal function after elective colonic resection: a randomised controlled trial. Lancet. 2002;359:1812–8.

14. Marjanovic G, Villain C, Juettner E, zur Hausen A, Hoeppner J, Hopt UT, et al. Impact of different crystalloid volume regimes on intestinal anastomotic stability. Ann Surg. 2009;249:181–5.

15. Nisanevich V, Felsenstein I, Almogy G, Weissman C, Einav S, Matot I. Effect of intraoperative fluid management on outcome after intraabdominal surgery. Anesthesiology. 2005;103:25–32.

16. McArdle GT, McAuley DF, McKinley A, Blair P, Hoper M, Harkin DW. Preliminary results of a prospective randomized trial of restrictive versus standard fluid regime in elective open abdominal aortic aneurysm repair. Ann Surg. 2009;250:28–34.

17. Rahbari NN, Zimmermann JB, Schmidt T, Koch M, Weigand MA, Weitz J. Meta-analysis of standard, restrictive and supplemental fluid administration in colorectal surgery. Br J Surg. 2009;96:331–41.

18. Lassen K, Soop M, Nygren J, Cox PB, Hendry PO, Spies C, et al. Consensus review of optimal perioperative care in colorectal surgery: Enhanced Recovery After Surgery (ERAS) Group recommendations. Arch Surg. 2009;144:961–9.

19. Lobo DN, Dube MG, Neal KR, Simpson J, Rowlands BJ, Allison SP. Problems with solutions: drowning in the brine of an inadequate knowledge base. Clin Nutr. 2001;20:125–30.

20. Stoneham MD, Hill EL. Variability in post-operative fluid and electrolyte prescription. Br J Clin Pract. 1997;51:82–4.

21. Lobo DN, Stanga Z, Aloysius MM, Wicks C, Nunes QM, Ingram KL, et al. Effect of volume loading with 1 liter intravenous infusions of 0.9% saline, 4% succinylated gelatine (Gelofusine) and 6% hydroxyethyl starch (Voluven) on blood volume and endocrine responses: a randomized, three-way crossover study in healthy volunteers. Crit Care Med. 2010;38:464–70.

22. Itobi E, Stroud M, Elia M. Impact of oedema on recovery after major abdominal surgery and potential value of multifrequency bioimpedance measurements. Br J Surg. 2006;93:354–61.

23. Awad S, Allison SP, Lobo DN. The history of 0.9% saline. Clin Nutr. 2008;27:179–88.

24. Lazarus-Barlow WS. On the initial rate of osmosis of blood-serum with reference to the composition of "physiological saline solution" in mammals. J Physiol. 1896;20:145–57.

25. Hamburger HJ. A discourse on permeability in physiology and pathology. Lancet. 1921;198:1039–45.

26. Veech RL. The toxic impact of parenteral solutions on the metabolism of cells: a hypothesis for physiological parenteral therapy. Am J Clin Nutr. 1986;44:519–51.

27. Wakim KG. 'Normal' 0.9 per cent salt solution is neither 'normal' nor physiological. JAMA. 1970;214:1710.

28. O'Malley CM, Frumento RJ, Hardy MA, Benvenisty AI, Brentjens TE, Mercer JS, et al. A randomized, double-blind comparison of lactated Ringer's solution and 0.9% NaCl during renal transplantation. Anesth Analg. 2005;100:1518–24.

29. Waters JH, Gottlieb A, Schoenwald P, Popovich MJ, Sprung J, Nelson DR. Normal saline versus lactated Ringer's solution for intraoperative fluid management in patients undergoing abdominal aortic aneurysm repair: an outcome study. Anesth Analg. 2001;93:817–22.

30. Ho AM, Karmakar MK, Contardi LH, Ng SS, Hewson JR. Excessive use of normal saline in managing traumatized patients in shock: a preventable contributor to acidosis. J Trauma. 2001;51:173–7.

31. Drummer C, Gerzer R, Heer M, Molz B, Bie P, Schlossberger M, et al. Effects of an acute saline infusion on fluid and electrolyte metabolism in humans. Am J Physiol. 1992;262: F744–54.
32. Lobo DN, Stanga Z, Simpson JAD, Anderson JA, Rowlands BJ, Allison SP. Dilution and redistribution effects of rapid 2-litre infusions of 0.9% (w/v) saline and 5% (w/v) dextrose on haematological parameters and serum biochemistry in normal subjects: a double-blind cross-over study. Clin Sci (Lond). 2001;101:173–9.
33. Reid F, Lobo DN, Williams RN, Rowlands BJ, Allison SP. (Ab)normal saline and physiological Hartmann's solution: a randomized double-blind crossover study. Clin Sci (Lond). 2003;104:17–24.
34. Moore FD. Metabolic care of the surgical patient. Philadelphia: W. B. Saunders; 1959.
35. Wilkinson AW, Billing BH, Nagy G, Stewart CP. Excretion of chloride and sodium after surgical operations. Lancet. 1949;1:640–4.
36. Gosling P. Salt of the earth or a drop in the ocean? A pathophysiological approach to fluid resuscitation. Emerg Med J. 2003;20:306–15.
37. Wilkes NJ, Woolf R, Mutch M, Mallett SV, Peachey T, Stephens R, et al. The effects of balanced versus saline-based hetastarch and crystalloid solutions on acid-base and electrolyte status and gastric mucosal perfusion in elderly surgical patients. Anesth Analg. 2001; 93:811–6.
38. Williams EL, Hildebrand KL, McCormick SA, Bedel MJ. The effect of intravenous lactated Ringer's solution versus 0.9% sodium chloride solution on serum osmolality in human volunteers. Anesth Analg. 1999;88:999–1003.
39. Wilcox CS. Regulation of renal blood flow by plasma chloride. J Clin Invest. 1983;71:726–35.
40. Matthay MA, Fukuda N, Frank J, Kallet R, Daniel B, Sakuma T. Alveolar epithelial barrier. Role in lung fluid balance in clinical lung injury. Clin Chest Med. 2000;21:477–90.
41. Wade CE, Grady JJ, Kramer GC, Younes RN, Gehlsen K, Holcroft JW. Individual patient cohort analysis of the efficacy of hypertonic saline/dextran in patients with traumatic brain injury and hypotension. J Trauma. 1997;42:S61–5.
42. Mecray PM, Barden RP, Ravdin IS. Nutritional edema: its effect on the gastric emptying time before and after gastric operations. Surgery. 1937;1:53–64.
43. Tournadre JP, Allaouchiche B, Malbert CH, Chassard D. Metabolic acidosis and respiratory acidosis impair gastro-pyloric motility in anesthetized pigs. Anesth Analg. 2000;90:74–9.
44. Mayberry JC, Welker KJ, Goldman RK, Mullins RJ. Mechanism of acute ascites formation after trauma resuscitation. Arch Surg. 2003;138:773–6.
45. Balogh Z, McKinley BA, Cocanour CS, Kozar RA, Valdivia A, Sailors RM, et al. Supranormal trauma resuscitation causes more cases of abdominal compartment syndrome. Arch Surg. 2003;138:637–42; discussion 642–3.
46. Macafee DA, Allison SP, Lobo DN. Some interactions between gastrointestinal function and fluid and electrolyte homeostasis. Curr Opin Clin Nutr Metab Care. 2005;8:197–203.
47. Holte K, Sharrock NE, Kehlet H. Pathophysiology and clinical implications of perioperative fluid excess. Br J Anaesth. 2002;89:622–32.
48. Cotton BA, Guy JS, Morris Jr JA. The cellular, metabolic, and systemic consequences of aggressive fluid resuscitation strategies. Shock. 2006;26:115–21.
49. Ringer S. Concerning the influence exerted by each of the constituents of the blood on the contraction of the ventricle. J Physiol. 1882;3:380–93.
50. Cushing H. Concerning the poisonous effect of pure sodium chloride solutions upon the nerve-muscle preparation. Am J Physiol. 1901;6:77–90.
51. Vermeulen H, Hofland J, Legemate DA, Ubbink DT. Intravenous fluid restriction after major abdominal surgery: a randomized blinded clinical trial. Trials. 2009;10:50.
52. Bellamy MC. Wet, dry or something else? Br J Anaesth. 2006;97:755–7.
53. Lobo DN, Allison SP. Fluid, electrolyte and nutrient replacement. In: Burnand KG, Young AE, Lucas J, Rowlands BJ, Scholefield J, editors. The new aird's companion in surgical studies. London: Churchill Livingstone; 2005. p. 20–41.
54. Mythen MG, Webb AR. Intra-operative gut mucosal hypoperfusion is associated with increased post-operative complications and cost. Intensive Care Med. 1994;20:99–104.

55. Kaye AD, Grogono AW. Fluid and electrolyte physiology. In: Miller RD, Cucchiara RF, Miller Jr ED, Reves JG, Roizen MF, Savarese JJ, editors. Anesthesia, vol. 1. Philadelphia: Churchill Livingstone; 2000. p. 1586–612.
56. Lamke LO, Liljedahl SO. Plasma volume changes after infusion of various plasma expanders. Resuscitation. 1976;5:93–102.
57. Svensen C, Hahn RG. Volume kinetics of Ringer solution, dextran 70, and hypertonic saline in male volunteers. Anesthesiology. 1997;87:204–12.
58. Lane N, Allen K. Hyponatraemia after orthopaedic surgery. BMJ. 1999;318:1363–4.
59. Nolan J. Fluid replacement. Br Med Bull. 1999;55:821–43.
60. Boldt J. Volume replacement in the surgical patient - does the type of solution make a difference? Br J Anaesth. 2000;84:783–93.
61. Hiltebrand LB, Kimberger O, Arnberger M, Brandt S, Kurz A, Sigurdsson GH. Crystalloids versus colloids for goal-directed fluid therapy in major surgery. Crit Care. 2009;13:R40.
62. Alderson P, Schierhout G, Roberts I, Bunn F. Colloids versus crystalloids for fluid resuscitation in critically ill patients. Cochrane Database Syst Rev. 2000;(2):CD000567.
63. Bunn F, Alderson P, Hawkins V. Colloid solutions for fluid resuscitation. Cochrane Database Syst Rev. 2000;(2):CD001319.
64. Choi PTL, Yip G, Quinonez LG, Cook DJ. Crystalloids vs. colloids in fluid resuscitation: a systematic review. Crit Care Med. 1999;27:200–10.
65. Perel P, Roberts I. Colloids versus crystalloids for fluid resuscitation in critically ill patients. Cochrane Database Syst Rev. 2007;(4):CD000567.
66. Senagore AJ, Emery T, Luchtefeld M, Kim D, Dujovny N, Hoedema R. Fluid management for laparoscopic colectomy: a prospective, randomized assessment of goal-directed administration of balanced salt solution or hetastarch coupled with an enhanced recovery program. Dis Colon Rectum. 2009;52:1935–40.
67. Bisonni RS, Holtgrave DR, Lawler F, Marley DS. Colloids versus crystalloids in fluid resuscitation - an analysis of randomized controlled trials. J Fam Pract. 1991;32:387–90.
68. Simmonds PD, Best L, George S, Baughan C, Buchanan R, Davis C, et al. Surgery for colorectal cancer in elderly patients: a systematic review. Colorectal Cancer Collaborative Group. Lancet 2000;356:968–74.
69. Desborough JP. The stress response to trauma and surgery. Br J Anaesth. 2000;85:109–17.
70. Alsous F, Khamiees M, DeGirolamo A, Amoateng-Adjepong Y, Manthous CA. Negative fluid balance predicts survival in patients with septic shock: a retrospective pilot study. Chest. 2000; 117:1749–54.
71. Joshi GP. Intraoperative fluid restriction improves outcome after major elective gastrointestinal surgery. Anesth Analg. 2005;101:601–5.
72. Holte K, Foss NB, Andersen J, Valentiner L, Lund C, Bie P, et al. Liberal or restrictive fluid administration in fast-track colonic surgery: a randomized, double-blind study. Br J Anaesth. 2007;99:500–8.
73. Gonzalez-Fajardo JA, Mengibar L, Brizuela JA, Castrodeza J, Vaquero-Puerta C. Effect of postoperative restrictive fluid therapy in the recovery of patients with abdominal vascular surgery. Eur J Vasc Endovasc Surg. 2009;37:538–43.
74. MacKay G, Fearon K, McConnachie A, Serpell MG, Molloy RG, O'Dwyer PJ. Randomized clinical trial of the effect of postoperative intravenous fluid restriction on recovery after elective colorectal surgery. Br J Surg. 2006;93:1469–74.
75. Kabon B, Akca O, Taguchi A, Nagele A, Jebadurai R, Arkilic CF, et al. Supplemental intravenous crystalloid administration does not reduce the risk of surgical wound infection. Anesth Analg. 2005;101:1546–53.
76. Lobo DN, Macafee DA, Allison SP. How perioperative fluid balance influences postoperative outcomes. Best Pract Res Clin Anaesthesiol. 2006;20:439–55.
77. Junghans T, Neuss H, Strohauer M, Raue W, Haase O, Schink T, et al. Hypovolemia after traditional preoperative care in patients undergoing colonic surgery is underrepresented in conventional hemodynamic monitoring. Int J Colorectal Dis. 2006;21:693–7.

78. Mowatt G, Houston G, Hernandez R, de Verteuil R, Fraser C, Cuthbertson B, et al. Systematic review of the clinical effectiveness and cost-effectiveness of oesophageal Doppler monitoring in critically ill and high-risk surgical patients. Health Technol Assess. 2009;13:iii–iv. ix–xii, 1–95.
79. Green D, Paklet L. Latest developments in peri-operative monitoring of the high-risk major surgery patient. Int J Surg. 2010;8:90–9.
80. Pearse R, Dawson D, Fawcett J, Rhodes A, Grounds RM, Bennett ED. Early goal-directed therapy after major surgery reduces complications and duration of hospital stay. A randomised, controlled trial [ISRCTN38797445]. Crit Care. 2005;9:R687–93.
81. Belloni L, Pisano A, Natale A, Piccirillo MR, Piazza L, Ismeno G, et al. Assessment of fluid-responsiveness parameters for off-pump coronary artery bypass surgery: a comparison among LiDCO, transesophageal echochardiography, and pulmonary artery catheter. J Cardiothorac Vasc Anesth. 2008;22:243–8.
82. Pearse RM, Ikram K, Barry J. Equipment review: an appraisal of the LiDCO plus method of measuring cardiac output. Crit Care. 2004;8:190–5.
83. Pittman J, Bar-Yosef S, SumPing J, Sherwood M, Mark J. Continuous cardiac output monitoring with pulse contour analysis: a comparison with lithium indicator dilution cardiac output measurement. Crit Care Med. 2005;33:2015–21.
84. Bundgaard-Nielsen M, Ruhnau B, Secher NH, Kehlet H. Flow-related techniques for preoperative goal-directed fluid optimization. Br J Anaesth. 2007;98:38–44.
85. Pearse RM, Rhodes A, Grounds RM. Clinical review: how to optimize management of high-risk surgical patients. Crit Care. 2004;8:503–7.
86. Noblett SE, Snowden CP, Shenton BK, Horgan AF. Randomized clinical trial assessing the effect of Doppler-optimized fluid management on outcome after elective colorectal resection. Br J Surg. 2006;93:1069–76.
87. Conway DH, Mayall R, Abdul-Latif MS, Gilligan S, Tackaberry C. Randomised controlled trial investigating the influence of intravenous fluid titration using oesophageal Doppler monitoring during bowel surgery. Anaesthesia. 2002;57:845–9.
88. Gan TJ, Soppitt A, Maroof M, el-Moalem H, Robertson KM, Moretti E, et al. Goal-directed intraoperative fluid administration reduces length of hospital stay after major surgery. Anesthesiology. 2002;97:820–6.
89. Wakeling HG, McFall MR, Jenkins CS, Woods WG, Miles WF, Barclay GR, et al. Intraoperative oesophageal Doppler guided fluid management shortens postoperative hospital stay after major bowel surgery. Br J Anaesth. 2005;95:634–42.
90. Donati A, Loggi S, Preiser JC, Orsetti G, Munch C, Gabbanelli V, et al. Goal-directed intraoperative therapy reduces morbidity and length of hospital stay in high-risk surgical patients. Chest. 2007;132:1817–24.
91. Boyd O, Grounds RM, Bennett ED. A randomized clinical trial of the effect of deliberate perioperative increase of oxygen delivery on mortality in high-risk surgical patients. JAMA. 1993;270:2699–707.
92. Shoemaker WC, Appel PL, Kram HB, Waxman K, Lee TS. Prospective trial of supranormal values of survivors as therapeutic goals in high-risk surgical patients. Chest. 1988;94:1176–86.
93. Wilson J, Woods I, Fawcett J, Whall R, Dibb W, Morris C, et al. Reducing the risk of major elective surgery: randomised controlled trial of preoperative optimisation of oxygen delivery. BMJ. 1999;318:1099–103.
94. Bundgaard-Nielsen M, Jorgensen CC, Secher NH, Kehlet H. Functional intravascular volume deficit in patients before surgery. Acta Anaesthesiol Scand. 2010;54:464–9.
95. Walsh SR, Tang T, Bass S, Gaunt ME. Doppler-guided intra-operative fluid management during major abdominal surgery: systematic review and meta-analysis. Int J Clin Pract. 2008;62:466–70.
96. Sinclair S, James S, Singer M. Intraoperative intravascular volume optimisation and length of hospital stay after repair of proximal femoral fracture: randomised controlled trial. BMJ. 1997;315:909–12.

97. Venn R, Steele A, Richardson P, Poloniecki J, Grounds M, Newman P. Randomized controlled trial to investigate influence of the fluid challenge on duration of hospital stay and perioperative morbidity in patients with hip fractures. Br J Anaesth. 2002;88:65–71.

98. Stone MD, Wilson RJ, Cross J, Williams BT. Effect of adding dopexamine to intraoperative volume expansion in patients undergoing major elective abdominal surgery. Br J Anaesth. 2003;91:619–24.

99. Davies SJ, Yates D, Wilson RJ. Dopexamine has no additional benefit in high-risk patients receiving goal-directed fluid therapy undergoing major abdominal surgery. Anesth Analg. 2011;112:130–8.

100. White PF, Kehlet H, Neal JM, Schricker T, Carr DB, Carli F. The role of the anesthesiologist in fast-track surgery: from multimodal analgesia to perioperative medical care. Anesth Analg. 2007;104:1380–96, table of contents.

101. Chung HM, Kluge R, Schrier RW, Anderson RJ. Clinical assessment of extracellular fluid volume in hyponatremia. Am J Med. 1987;83:905–8.

102. Bamboat ZM, Bordeianou L. Perioperative fluid management. Clin Colon Rectal Surg. 2009;22:28–33.

103. Holte K, Nielsen KG, Madsen JL, Kehlet H. Physiologic effects of bowel preparation. Dis Colon Rectum. 2004;47:1397–402.

104. Guenaga KF, Matos D, Castro AA, Atallah AN, Wille-Jorgensen P. Mechanical bowel preparation for elective colorectal surgery. Cochrane Database Syst Rev. 2005;(1):CD001544.

105. Platell C, Hall J. What is the role of mechanical bowel preparation in patients undergoing colorectal surgery? Dis Colon Rectum. 1998;41:875–82; discussion 882–3.

106. Ram E, Sherman Y, Weil R, Vishne T, Kravarusic D, Dreznik Z. Is mechanical bowel preparation mandatory for elective colon surgery? A prospective randomized study. Arch Surg. 2005;140:285–8.

107. Jung B, Pahlman L, Nystrom PO, Nilsson E. Multicentre randomized clinical trial of mechanical bowel preparation in elective colonic resection. Br J Surg. 2007;94:689–95.

108. Slim K, Vicaut E, Panis Y, Chipponi J. Meta-analysis of randomized clinical trials of colorectal surgery with or without mechanical bowel preparation. Br J Surg. 2004;91:1125–30.

109. Sanders G, Arthur CH, Hosie KB, Lambert AW. Is patient outcome affected by the administration of intravenous fluid during bowel preparation for colonic surgery? Ann R Coll Surg Engl. 2007;89:487–9.

110. Thorell A, Nygren J, Ljungqvist O. Insulin resistance: a marker of surgical stress. Curr Opin Clin Nutr Metab Care. 1999;2:69–78.

111. Thorell A, Efendic S, Gutniak M, Haggmark T, Ljungqvist O. Development of postoperative insulin resistance is associated with the magnitude of operation. Eur J Surg. 1993;159:593–9.

112. Hendry PO, Balfour A, Potter MA, Mander BJ, Bartolo DC, Anderson DN, et al. Preoperative conditioning with oral carbohydrate loading and oral nutritional supplements can be combined with mechanical bowel preparation prior to elective colorectal resection. Colorectal Dis. 2008;10:907–10.

113. Brady M, Kinn S, Stuart P. Preoperative fasting for adults to prevent perioperative complications. Cochrane Database Syst Rev. 2003;(4):CD004423.

114. Starker PM, Lasala PA, Askanazi J, Gump FE, Forse RA, Kinney JM. The response to TPN. A form of nutritional assessment. Ann Surg. 1983;198:720–4.

115. Gil MJ, Franch G, Guirao X, Oliva A, Herms R, Salas E, et al. Response of severely malnourished patients to preoperative parenteral nutrition: a randomized clinical trial of water and sodium restriction. Nutrition. 1997;13:26–31.

116. Arieff AI. Fatal postoperative pulmonary edema: pathogenesis and literature review. Chest. 1999;115:1371–7.

117. Tambyraja AL, Sengupta F, MacGregor AB, Bartolo DC, Fearon KC. Patterns and clinical outcomes associated with routine intravenous sodium and fluid administration after colorectal resection. World J Surg. 2004;28:1046–51; discussion 1051–2.
118. Lowell JA, Schifferdecker C, Driscoll DF, Benotti PN, Bistrian BR. Postoperative fluid overload: not a benign problem. Crit Care Med. 1990;18:728–33.
119. Miedema BW, Johnson JO. Methods for decreasing postoperative gut dysmotility. Lancet Oncol. 2003;4:365–72.
120. Rusch D, Eberhart L, Biedler A, Dethling J, Apfel CC. Prospective application of a simplified risk score to prevent postoperative nausea and vomiting. Can J Anaesth. 2005;52:478–84.
121. Apfel CC, Kranke P, Eberhart LH, Roos A, Roewer N. Comparison of predictive models for postoperative nausea and vomiting. Br J Anaesth. 2002;88:234–40.
122. Carlisle JB, Stevenson CA. Drugs for preventing postoperative nausea and vomiting. Cochrane Database Syst Rev. 2006;(3): CD004125.
123. Wallenborn J, Gelbrich G, Bulst D, Behrends K, Wallenborn H, Rohrbach A, et al. Prevention of postoperative nausea and vomiting by metoclopramide combined with dexamethasone: randomised double blind multicentre trial. BMJ. 2006;333:324.
124. Nelson R, Edwards S, Tse B. Prophylactic nasogastric decompression after abdominal surgery. Cochrane Database Syst Rev. 2007;(3): CD004929.
125. Andersen HK, Lewis SJ, Thomas S. Early enteral nutrition within 24 h of colorectal surgery versus later commencement of feeding for postoperative complications. Cochrane Database Syst Rev. 2006: CD004080.
126. Holte K, Foss NB, Svensen C, Lund C, Madsen JL, Kehlet H. Epidural anesthesia, hypotension, and changes in intravascular volume. Anesthesiology. 2004;100:281–6.

Chapter 6
Pain Control After Surgery

William J. Fawcett

Introduction

Good pain control following surgery is a cornerstone of modern perioperative care. Aside from the humanitarian considerations, good pain control should allow patients to mobilise more swiftly, lessen organ dysfunction, begin earlier nutrition and ultimately allow quicker discharge home [1]. Within the context of enhanced recovery (ER), various pain control modalities may also have secondary effects on the physiological response to surgery and fluid administration. Thus pain control should be viewed not in isolation but as hopefully promoting and certainly not hindering other aspects of ER.

The two fundamental areas to consider are the analgesic drugs themselves and the route of their administration.

Analgesic Drugs

There are many different drugs available for pain control (Table 6.1). Opioids are the principal drugs for postoperative pain, of which morphine is viewed the gold standard. Whilst morphine provides effective pain relief it has many adverse effects, some of which are particularly relevant to colorectal surgery. The major focus in the last two decades has therefore been to add to analgesics different mechanisms of action so that there is a morphine-sparing effect. This concept of multi-modal or balanced analgesia minimises opioid use whilst still permitting good overall pain control.

W.J. Fawcett
Department of Anaesthesia, Royal Surrey County Hospital NHS Foundation Trust,
Guildford, Surrey, UK

N. Francis et al. (eds.), *Manual of Fast Track Recovery for Colorectal Surgery*,
Enhanced Recovery, DOI 10.1007/978-0-85729-953-6_6,
© Springer-Verlag London Limited 2012

Table 6.1 Drugs used to control pain

Opioids agonist, e.g. morphine, pethidine, diamorphine, codeine
Local anaesthetics, e.g. bupivacaine, lidocaine
Anti-inflammatory drugs
Traditional NSAIDS. e.g. diclofenac and ibuprofen
Selective cyclooxygenase (COX)-type 2 inhibitors, e.g. parecoxib
Paracetamol
Miscellenaeous
Tramadol (opioid agonist and noradrenaline and serotonin
  reuptake inhibitor)
NMDA receptor antagonists, e.g. ketamine and magnesium
Anti-convulsants, e.g. pregablin, gabapentin
Alpha-2 agonists, e.g. clonidine

Routes of Administration

Getting analgesic drugs rapidly and in the correct concentration to the site of action is essential for good pain control. Intravenous administration gives rapid plasma levels and for patients undergoing surgery, this method is practical and generally effective. The oral route may be effective, but will require absorption from the gastrointestinal tract. In addition, some drugs, for example opioids, have a significant first pass effect and the oral dose needs to be increased to allow for this.

Other routes commonly used are rectal (not suitable for low rectal anastomoses), intramuscular and more rarely transdermal and intranasal. Both local anaesthetics and opioids can be administered via the spinal and epidural route. In addition, local anaesthetics can be given as local nerve blocks.

In addition to the use of these drugs, if patients are going to benefit fully from an ER programme, then they will need access to an acute pain service, which with the ward staff can undertake careful documenting of pain problems, sedation, respiratory rate and other parameters and, where necessary, intervene to correct problems.

Classical Approach to Analgesia for Colorectal Surgery

Epidural Analgesia (Extradural)

The widespread introduction of epidural analgesia for open colorectal surgery has had a dramatic effect on the postoperative course. Both local anaesthetics and opioids may be used, but they are most commonly used together. Whilst providing superlative segmental pain relief, epidurals also have other physiological effects (Table 6.2) in particular a degree of sympathetic nerve blockade leading to hypotension. There is commonly interference with bladder emptying, and in addition any opioid used may have systemic effects such as respiratory depression, itching and postoperative nausea and vomiting (PONV).

Table 6.2 Effects of neuraxial anaesthesia (epidural and spinal)

Local anaesthetic
Sensory nerves
Pain relief
Numbness
Loss of proprioception
Urinary retention
Motor nerves
Muscle weakness
Urinary retention
Sympathetic nerves
Hypotension
Bradycardia
Opioid
Respiratory depression
Drowsiness
Itching
Urinary retention
PONV

The effects of epidurals have been well studied for 20 years and several meta-analyses have provided encouraging results for the use of epidurals in major surgery. Rodgers' paper examined 141 trials with 9,559 patients from New Zealand and is typical where a dramatic reduction in mortality (30%), deep vein thrombosis (44%), pulmonary embolism (55%), blood transfusion requirements (50%), pneumonia (39%) and respiratory depression (59%) were shown [2].

Of particular relevance to patients undergoing colorectal surgery is the return to normal GI function so that enteral feeding can be resumed. Thus any prolongation of a postoperative ileus is most detrimental. The use of opioids is a major factor here and several studies have convincingly shown that the use of continuous epidural infusion with local anaesthetic compared to opioid is very effective at reducing postoperative ileus.

However, there are numerous problems with epidurals and some studies have shown epidurals to be much less effective than previously thought: Indeed the MASTER Trial (in which 915 high-risk patients in Australia undergoing major abdominal surgery were randomised to receive an epidural or alternative regimes) showed a trend towards increasing mortality – 5.1% vs 4.3% with no difference in morbidity [3]. More recently the focus for potential harm that can arise from epidurals is gaining momentum. Common problems include epidural failure, hypotension, poor mobility and permanent neurological damage.

An ineffective epidural is a common and serious problem, occurring in up to 50% of patients. Often the patient is in pain for several hours whilst the attempts are made to top up the epidural, position the patient differently, etc. and sometimes all to avail. In addition, whilst a local anaesthetic/opioid infusion is in progress, the patient cannot receive other opioids.

Hypotension is a significant issue too especially for colorectal surgery. Anastomotic healing appears to be dependent on blood pressure and efforts have to

Table 6.3 Stress response to surgery

Endocrine activation (pituitary and adrenals)
Increase in cortisol, growth hormone, aldosterone, glucagon, ADH
Sympathetic system activation (epinephrine and norepinephrine)
Reduction in insulin
Metabolic consequences
Protein catabolism, lipolysis, hyperglycaemia, salt and water retention
Inflammatory mediator activation
Cytokines, e.g. interleukin-6
Immunosuppression
Reduced cell-mediated immunity

be taken to ensure this is effective. The problem is that treating patient with further i.v. fluids, often almost a reflex response by junior medical staff in these patients, may involve the ultimate administration of several litres of excess fluid and saline, which is counter-productive to all patients especially those in whom enhanced recovery is contemplated. This has detrimental effects not only on the anastomosis but also in patients at risk of myocardial ischaemia and pulmonary oedema. In addition excess i.v. fluids can prolong the paralytic ileus and cause electrolyte disturbances and may decrease tissue oxygenation and affect anastomotic healing [4].

Mobilisation postoperatively for patients with epidural infusions is sometimes a problem. Depending on the rate and concentration of bupivicaine (typically between 0.1% and 0.15%), there may be an element of motor block and of loss of proprioception. This together with potentially a significant postural element to the blood pressure (vide supra), and occasionally other factors such as poor nurse-to-patient ratio and lack of familiarity of epidurals by ward staff can sometimes mean patients are unnecessarily confined to bed rest whilst an epidural is running.

Neurological damage and death, although rare, still needs to be considered with permanent injury occurring in the ratio of 1:24,000–1:54,000 and death/paraplegia in 1:50,000–1:140,000 cases.

Finally another area involving epidurals involves the stress response to surgery. This is a systemic change following surgery and trauma and involves a number of physiological sequelae (Table 6.3).

These effects are magnified by starvation, infection and hypovolaemia. Although avoidance of the stress response is seen as desirable, especially within the ER setting, its modification is still, disappointingly, generally of unproven benefit. However within ER, efforts are nevertheless made to reduce the stress response by other mechanisms and include careful attention to fluid therapy, preoperative carbohydrate loading and early enteral feeding.

To date, the majority of data has been collected on patients undergoing traditional open surgery. Therefore the crucial question is this 'How much of the above in transferable to ER, and in particular to minimal access surgery?' There are some key differences:

- Intraoperative cardiopulmonary stresses are greater and effects of block magnified during laparoscopic colorectal surgery.

- Steep positioning and pneumoperitoneum can affect block height.
- Abdominal incision is smaller, transverse and below the umbilicus.
- There may be shoulder tip pain from laparoscopy.
- Analgesic requirements at 24 h can usually be addressed with simple analgesics.

Although historically a mid-thoracic epidural is viewed almost as a pre-requisite in ER, many regard it as unnecessary and even meddlesome, as overall pain relief requirements are less compared to open surgery. Moreover, it will not effectively treat shoulder pain, may impair mobilisation and adversely affect fluid balance. Some have found epidurals to be effective, but there is a growing acceptance that this mode of analgesia may simply not be warranted for patients undergoing laparoscopic bowel resection.

Other Approaches to Pain Control

If epidurals, once the mainstay of analgesia for open colorectal surgery, have a lesser role in minimal access surgery, then other therapeutic options need to be assessed.

Spinal Anaesthesia (Subarachnoid or Intrathecal)

Spinal anaesthesia, whilst having many of the attributes of epidural blockade, is not generally extendable into the postoperative period via a catheter as it is a single-shot approach. Generally this technique is not suitable for open surgery whereby intensive pain relief is required for 48 h or more. However, for minimal access surgery where pain relief requirements are modest by the second postoperative day, they are logical and we used them with good effect for 23-h stay laparoscopic colectomy [5, 6].

As with epidurals, many use a combination of local anaesthesia (0.5% bupivicaine) and an opioid. Diamorphine, which is commonly used in obstetrics, provides predictable, safe and effective analgesia in a dose-dependent fashion postoperatively. A dose of 0.25 mg, extrapolated from obstetrics, provides analgesia for 7–8 h postoperatively [7]. Higher doses extend both the duration of analgesia but also opioid-related adverse effects.

Although spinals may produce reduced blood loss, pulmonary thromboemboli and a temporary marked reduction in various aspects of the stress response, with increase in sympathetic tone to the gut, there are a number of key general differences compared to epidurals (Table 6.4). In addition, with particular relevance to patients undergoing laparoscopic colorectal resection, there are specific differences including

- Risk of exaggerated cardiovascular changes
- Risk of high block, particularly during head down positioning
- Postoperative mobilisation improved

Table 6.4 Comparison of epidurals and spinals

Epidural	Spinal
High volume required, e.g. 20–25 mL	Low volume, e.g. 3 mL
Catheter inserted: extendable for several days	Single shot (only last hours)
Slow onset	Rapid onset
May get missed segments	Usually very effective
More difficult technique	Easier technique
Identifying epidural space	Simple end point
Positioning catheter	Higher success rate
High complication rate	Lower complication rate

If spinals are to be used for ER patients, especially with laparoscopic surgery then patients need at least 20 min for the block to fix prior to be positioned head down. From our randomised controlled trial comparing spinals, epidurals or patient-controlled analgesia (PCA) [8], evidence is accumulating that spinals result in

- Pain scores similar to epidurals with both better than PCA
- Need for vasoconstrictors less than epidurals
- Better preservation of respiratory compared to PCA
- Good opioid sparing effects
- Less postoperative fluids required and thus reduced weight gain than epidurals
- Urinary catheter removed more quickly than epidurals
- Reduced length of stay

Spinal anaesthesia seems to provide many of the intraoperative advantages of epidurals, yet due to their short action, avoid many of the postoperative disadvantages of epidurals, especially hypotension and poor mobilisation. By the time their effect is waning, it is reasonable to expect the patient's analgesia might be catered for by simple analgesics.

Other Local Anaesthetic Blocks

Anaesthetists may decide that the central blockade may be unnecessary, but the use of local anaesthetic peripherally should always be encouraged. There are a number of ways in which this can be achieved.

Transversus Abdominis Plane (TAP) Block

Given that a significant amount of pain from abdominal surgery comes from the abdominal wall incision, it is logical to assume that blockade of the neural afferents would be an effective method of postoperative analgesia. With TAP block, often with ultrasound guidance, local anaesthetic is injected into the neurofascial plane between the external oblique and the tranversus abdominis muscle in the triangle of

Petit. This can provide effective and reliable block for patients undergoing open abdominal surgery, with morphine requirements reduced by nearly 75% [9] in a study from Ireland where 32 patients were randomised to receive either PCA or TAP block. Another paper from Saudi Arabia reported that 42 patients were randomised to receive either TAP block or nothing, followed by PCA when undergoing laparoscopic surgery, also had a marked, albeit less, morphine-sparing effect (50% reduction) [10]. This technique is safe and has a promising role in the management of pain relief for patients within ER, although there is a recent report of liver damage following attempted ultrasound-guided TAP block [11].

Local Anaesthetic into Incision

Infiltration of the wound site by the surgeon should always be used if local anaesthetic has not been used previously. This approach is useful for several hours and can reduce early pain scores. A more logical approach is the use of a device to give a constant infusion of local anaesthetic into the wound for several days postoperatively. The device provides a continuous infusion via an elastomeric reservoir of local anaesthetic attached to a multi-holed catheter that lies along the length of the wound. It has been used for many types of surgery including thoracic, abdominal and pelvic surgery, as well as breast reconstruction and joint replacement surgery. There is some success with the device, reducing morphine requirements and pain scores, especially in the early postoperative period. One randomised placebo-controlled trial on 310 patients from Australia undergoing colorectal surgery demonstrated reduced pain scores in the first day but no advantage thereafter [12]. A recent meta-analysis of five trials with 542 laparotomy wounds confirmed its promise at reducing VAS and opioid consumption but without reducing length of stay or return of bowel function [13]. There is little evidence following minimal access surgery but a recent retrospective analysis of 38 patients from the United States did show a reduction in morphine use and hospital length of stay following laparoscopic renal surgery [14].

In summary, local anaesthetics are fundamental in delivering multi-modal analgesia. There are few patients who are unsuitable for local anaesthesia administered by one of the above routes.

Opioids

Strong Opioids

The majority of data relates to morphine. A fundamental prerequisite of analgesia is the avoidance of opioids where possible and indeed many studies give as their end point the 'opioid-sparing effect'. Traditionally, many regard the return of bowel function to be the rate-limiting factor in reducing length of stay in hospital and the role that morphine consumption has in this process. For example, Cali et al. showed a strong correlation in 40 patients between morphine consumption and return of bowel function, and in their study, no correlation was demonstrated between morphine consumption and wound length, concluding that efforts should be directed more towards diminishing use opioids than attempting to minimise abdominal incisions [15].

However, it is probably too simplistic to attribute hospital length of stay to be governed solely by the length of ileus as there are probably several other factors as well: Indeed it has been demonstrated that whilst epidurals had a marked opioid sparing effect and reduced ileus, length of time in hospital was slightly *increased* in the epidural group [16].

The advent of small incision/laparoscopic surgery, in spite of Cali's paper [15], is widely regarded as a big advance in reducing the length of stay and fundamental to ER. It is reasonable to expect ER patients to have a reduction in analgesic requirements, and so therefore if they do require opioids it will be for a shorter length of time and with less concomitant sequelae. Indeed this has been borne out by one of the few studies comparing PCA in 38 patients undergoing either laparoscopy or traditional laparotomy for bowel resection, with the former group having a more rapid hospital discharge. Interestingly bowel movements resumed earlier in the laparoscopic group with no relationship to morphine consumption and return of bowel function. Moreover, cumulative morphine consumption during the first two postoperative days was similar in both groups [17].

This suggests that morphine is no longer the sole villain within ER programmes. The ability of patients to participate successfully within the programme is multifactorial and whilst it is reasonable to limit where possible morphine and other strong opioids, their moderate use probably has less overall effect on outcome than previously thought. Furthermore, the reluctance to administer adequate pain relief to patients who are in pain is wrong and will not reduce their length of stay.

Weaker Opioids

There are a number of commonly used weaker opioids including codeine and tramadol. Codeine is metabolised via several pathways, with morphine as one of the metabolites. It is well known to cause constipation but is still a commonly used drug when pain requirements are modest. Perhaps a more logical drug is tramadol, which not only has agonist activity at μ-opioid receptors but also inhibits reuptake of norepinephrine and serotonin. However it still has the expected side effects including nausea, vomiting, constipation and dypshoria. It has been used intravenously (including PCA), intramuscularly and orally. Generally codeine or tramadol are most useful orally with ER programmes after 24 h as pain relief requirements reduce.

A new drug of relevance to the use of opioids is alvimopan, which is a novel class of drug. It is a peripherally acting μ-opioid receptor antagonist and is designed to reverse opioid-induced side effects on the gastrointestinal system without compromising on centrally mediated pain relief. Early studies in its use are promising although there is some association with an increased rate of myocardial infarction [18].

Non-steroidal Anti-inflammatory Drugs (NSAIDS) and Selective Cyclooxygenase (COX) Type 2 Inhibitors

These drugs play a key role in ER. They have a well-documented opioid-sparing effect and are a key component of multi-modal analgesia. Given the cascade of activation that occurs following surgery with release of cytokines and prostaglandins via cyclo-oxygenase (COX) activation, the COX inhibitors are logical agents to reduce inflammation and pain.

The traditional NSAIDs such as ibuprofen, diclofenac and ketorolac have a marked effect in reducing opioid consumption. Chen et al. showed a 30% reduction in opioid consumption and some improvement in overall bowel function in 79 patients but overall there was no consistent reduction in the length of postoperative ileus, suggesting that ileus is multifactorial and not just due to opioid consumption [19].

The selective COX-2 inhibitors have the advantage of a reduction in side effects associated with NSAIDs, particularly gastrointestinal side effects. Again there is an impressive reduction in opioid consumption – again by about a third – and with reduction in ileus [20].

The well-known side effects of NSAIDs are well known and include gastrointestinal bleeding, renal dysfunction, increased bleeding and allergies. In particular the risk of renal impairment is increased further in those patients with pre-existing renal dysfunction, hypovolaemaia and the concomitant use of other nephrotoxic drugs. Many units also try to minimise the risk of gastric erosions by the use of proton pump inhibitors. Recently reports have arisen from both classes of these drugs, suggesting an increase in anastomotic leakage and further work is required in this area [21, 22]. Finally although caution is required in the long-term use of COX-2 in patients at risk of cardiovascular events, they are probably safe for 3–5 days postoperatively [23].

In summary these classes of drugs remain an important aspect of multi-modal analgesia, but as other non-opioid agents are introduced (see later) their role may diminish somewhat. Moreover some have questioned the cost effectiveness of COX-2 inhibitors, arguing that traditional NSAIDs and paracetamol may be as effective.

Paracetamol

This drug is widely used in almost every multi-modal regime. Although only suitable for mild to moderate pain, it is, if correctly used, a safe drug and can be used alongside other analgesics. It is an entirely separate agent to the traditional NSAIDs and COX-2, having a central action probably mediated via stimulation of serotonergic pathways within the spinal cord, probably through enhancing the activity of cannabinoid receptors [24]. Like the NSAIDs, it has a significant though probably lesser opioid-sparing effect, but both drugs are probably superior in combination to either drug alone [25, 26]. The advent of intravenous paracetamol has enabled patients to receive appropriate dosing in throughout the perioperative period, unaffected by unreliable oral or rectal administration.

Alternative Approaches

There are many alternative approaches to the multi-modal concept of pain control. These include i.v. lidocaine, ketamine, oral pregabalin, magnesium, glucocorticoids and beta-blockers.

Lidocaine Infusions

Intravenous lidocaine was described over 50 years ago as an analgesic. More recently these analgesic properties have been confirmed, as well as anti-inflammatory and anti-hyperalgesic properties. These effects have recently been the subject of a meta-analysis [27] from France where eight trials and 161 patients were analysed who had received intravenous lidocaine, compared to 159 control patients. There were convincing reductions in pain relief requirements, ileus, PONV and length of stay. Another paper evaluated its use for laparoscopic colectomy and demonstrated that opioid consumption was reduced by two-thirds, with improved bowel function, less fatigue and a reduced hospital stay with endocrine and metabolic responses unchanged [28]. However, more recently the place of lidocaine infusions has been questioned in less major surgery. It may be that although i.v. lidocaine has significant effects for major and in particular open surgery, this effect may not translate to smaller incision surgery. Overall, though, it is a promising and evolving area.

Ketamine

Ketamine, which is an anaesthetic and analgesic agent, at low doses also improves analgesia, reduces morphine consumption and PONV with little in the way of attributable side effects. One of the problems associated with morphine and other opioid administration is acute tolerance and delayed hyperalgesia. These effects are mediated by at NMDA glutamate receptors and these effects are blocked by ketamine (an NMDA antagonist). The dose and duration of ketamine is still debated but in a recent study, when ketamine was used intraoperatively and postoperatively as an infusion for 48 h, the morphine consumption was nearly halved. Although ketamine has a number of side effects including sedation, delusions, nightmares and psychiatric disorders, these effects were not manifest at low doses of ketamine [29].

Magnesium

Given that ketamine is an NMDA antagonist, it is logical to assume that another antagonist at this receptor, extracellular magnesium, would confer some analgesia. This is indeed the case but the results are less impressive than with ketamine. Magnesium has been administered via a number of routes – intravenously, into the wound, intraarticular and epidurally. In addition timing, dose and duration are important in achieving its effects. Some studies have shown no discernible benefit, whilst some have shown some benefit with reduced opioid consumption. In addition it also improves postoperative analgesia in patients undergoing spinal analgesia. Magnesium has a number of other effects including muscle weakness and caution is required in its use [30].

Pregabalin

This agent and its developmental precursor, gabapentin, possess analgesic, anticonvulsant and anxiolytic effects and are commonly used in chronic pain. Whilst it might be expected to prevent the progression of acute pain to chronic pain, a few studies have found it useful for reduction in postoperative opioid analgesia requirements [31], whereas other have found it less useful. Moreover it has numerous side effects including sedation and confusion, which will probably limit its place within the ER setting [32]. The effects – both beneficial and harmful – may well be related to dose.

Others

Beta-blockers, whilst not analgesics, may be useful in the management of cardiovascular sequelae of poorly controlled pain. The POISE trial, a multinational study of 8,331 patients, demonstrated however that strokes and death were considerably increased in the beta-blocker (metoprolol) group [33], an effect possibly related to the dose. Currently, as a universal treatment, their usefulness is unknown and may indeed be harmful.

Glucocorticoids (e.g. dexamethasone) are commonly prescribed in the perioperative period for its anti-inflammatory and anti-emetic actions. There is some evidence that they reduce analgesic requirements and in addition may, like pregabalin, reduce the progression to chronic pain.

Practical Approach to the Management of Pain
for ER Patients (Table 6.5)

Table 6.5 (a) Analgesia for first 48 h (including anti-emetics and gastric mucosal protection) for both open and laparoscopic surgery

Preoperative medication	Postoperative regular medication	Postoperative rescue medication
Local anaesthetic Open surgery: Epidural or TAP block Lap. surgery: spinal/TAP block/wound infiltration	*Local anaesthetic* Open surgery: Epidural infusion or continuous wound infiltration	*Tramadol* 50–100 mg oral or intravenously 6 hourly (if not receiving it already)
Remifentanil infusion	*Paracetamol* 1 g oral or intravenously 6 hourly	*Morphine* Up to 10 mg intramuscularly or intravenously
Paracetamol 1 g i.v. 15 min prior to end of surgery	*Diclofenac* 50 mg oral 8 hourly once eating OR *Tramadol* 50–100 mg oral 6 hourly if diclofenac contraindicated	*Cyclizine* 25 mg intramuscularly or intravenously 6 hourly
Ondansetron 4 mg prior to end of surgery	*Omeprazole* 20 mg oral daily (with diclofenac)	*Ondansetron* 4 mg intravenously 6 hourly

Table 6.5 (b) Open surgery days 2–4

Regular medication	Rescue medication
Paracetamol 1 g oral or intravenously 6 hourly	*Tramadol* 50–100 mg oral or intravenously 6 hourly (if not receiving it already)
Diclofenac 50 mg oral 8 hourly once eating	*Morphine* Up to 10 mg intramuscularly or intravenously
Omeprazole 20 mg oral daily (with diclofenac)	*Cyclizine* 25 mg intramuscularly or intravenously 6 hourly
Tramadol 50–100 mg oral 6 hourly if diclofenac is contraindicated	*Ondansetron* 4 mg intravenously 6 hourly

Table 6.5 (c) Laparoscopic surgery days 2–4 and open surgery days 5–6

Regular medication
Paracetamol 1 g oral or intravenously 6 hourly
Diclofenac 50 mg oral 8 hourly
Tramadol 50–100 mg oral 6 hourly if diclofenac is contraindicated

Key points are:

- Starting simple analgesics (paracetamol and NSAIDs) early and regularly.
- Prescribing anti-emetics is essential. They are more effective when used in combination with the drugs possessing different mechanisms of action, such as cyclizine and ondansetron.
- If opioids are to be administered then the PCA morphine is popular, but any opioid-sparing procedure such as the use of lidocaine or magnesium should be considered.
- Patients should be monitored for side effects such from NSAIDs (gastrointestinal and renal), tramadol (PONV and sedation) or codeine (constipation).
- Patients differ markedly in how the drugs affect them both in terms of side effects and efficacy. Drugs should be substituted if they are not beneficial or cause unwanted effects.
- When considering drugs for discharge, patients may have their own supply of simple analgesics at home. They should be advised to take these regularly up to the maximum limits for paracetamol and NSAIDs. The use of co-drugs is common, e.g. cocodamol, but patients should be warned that they cannot take paracetamol concurrently. The use of regular analgesics for at least 72 h is advised.

Summary

Whilst good analgesia is fundamental for all patients undergoing major surgery it is not the only objective. For example, if the method chosen results in adverse effects (e.g. hypotension) and therefore excess fluid administration (e.g. regional blockade), excessive PONV or sedation, then the overall benefit for an ER patients may be negligible. Evidence is limited for laparoscopic/small incision surgery and extrapolating analgesic regimens from classical open surgery to ER patients may be unreliable. Whilst there are a number of promising drugs to add to the concept of multi-modal anaesthesia, the regular use of safe simple analgesics is vital. If pain control is problematic in the early operative period, the judicious use of morphine will almost always be required along with anti-emetics. If patients are to benefit fully from an enhanced recovery programme, then they must have regular input from a pain team as well as ensuring that the analgesic technique itself does not contribute to other problems and ultimately an increased length of stay in hospital.

References

1. Kehlet H. Fast track colorectal surgery. Lancet. 2008;371:791–3.
2. Rodgers A, Walker N, Schug S, McKee A, Kehlet H, van Zundert A, et al. Reduction of postoperative mortality and morbidity with epidural or spinal anaesthesia: results from overview of randomised trials. BMJ. 2000;321:1493.

3. Rigg JR, Jamrozik K, Myles PS, Silbert BS, Peyton PJ, Parsons RW, et al. Epidural anaesthesia and analgesia and outcome of major surgery: a randomised trial. Lancet. 2002;359:1276–82.
4. Holte K, Sharrock NE, Kehlet H. Pathophysiology and clinical implications of perioperative fluid excess. Br J Anaesth. 2002;89:622–32.
5. Levy BF, Tilney HS, Dowson HMP, Rockall TA. A systematic review of postoperative analgesia following laparoscopic colorectal surgery. Colorectal Dis. 2009;12:5–15.
6. Levy BF, Scott MJP, Fawcett WJ, Rockall TA. 23-Hour-Stay Laparoscopic Colectomy. Dis Colon Rectum. 2009;52:1239–43.
7. Saravanan S, Robinson APC, Qayoum Dar A, Columb MO, Lyons GR. Minimum dose of intrathecal diamorphine required to prevent intraoperative supplementation of spinal anaesthesia for Caesarean section. Br J Anaesth. 2003;91:368–72.
8. Levy BF, Fawcett WJ, Scott MJP, Rockall TA. Oxygen delivery in fluid optimised laparoscopic colorectal surgery with different analgesic modalities. (ASGBI ASM, Glasgow 2009). Br J Surg. 2009;96(S4):2–3.
9. McDonnell JG, O'Donnell B, Curley G, Heffernan A, Power C, Laffey JG. The analgesic efficacy of transversus abdominis plane block after abdominal surgery: a prospective randomized controlled trial. Anesth Analg. 2007;104:193–7.
10. El-Dawlatly AA, Turkistani A, Kettner SC, Machata A-M, Delvi MB, Thallaj A, et al. Ultrasound-guided transversus abdominis plane block: description of a new technique and comparison with conventional systemic analgesia during laparoscopic cholecystectomy. Br J Anaesth. 2009;102:763–7.
11. Lancaster P, Chadwick M. Liver trauma secondary to ultrasound guided transversus abdominis plane block. Br J Anaesth. 2010;104:509–10.
12. Polglase AL, McMurrick P, Simpson PJB, Wale RJ, Carne PWG, Johnson W, et al. Continuous wound infusion of local anesthetic for the control of pain after elective abdominal colorectal surgery. Dis Colon Rectum. 2007;50:2158–67.
13. Karthikesalingam A, Walsh SR, Markar SR, Sadat U, Tang TY, Malata CM. Continuous wound infusion of local anaesthetic agents following colorectal surgery: systematic review and meta-analysis. World J Gastroenterol. 2008;14:5301.
14. Yoost TR, McIntyre M, Savage SJ. Continuous infusion of local anesthetic decreases narcotic use and length of hospitalization after laparoscopic renal surgery. J Endourol. 2009;23:623–6.
15. Cali RL, Meade PG, Swanson MS, Freeman C. Effect of morphine and incision length on bowel function after colectomy. Dis Colon Rectum. 2000;43:163–8.
16. Carli F, Trudel JL, Belliveau P. The effect of intraoperative thoracic epidural anesthesia and postoperative analgesia on bowel function after colorectal surgery. Dis Colon Rectum. 2001;44:1083–9.
17. Hong X, Mistraletti G, Zandi S, Stein B, Charlebois P, Carli F. Laparoscopy for colectomy accelerates restoration of bowel function when using patient controlled analgesia. Can J Anesth. 2006;53:544–50.
18. Becker G, Blum H. Novel opioid antagonists for opioid-induced bowel dysfunction and postoperative ileus. Lancet. 2009;373:1198–206.
19. Chen JY, Wu GJ, Mok MS, Chou YH, Sun WZ, Chen PL, et al. Effect of adding ketorolac to intravenous morphine patient-controlled analgesia on bowel function in colorectal surgery patients–a prospective, randomized, double-blind study. Acta Anaesthesiol Scand. 2005;49:546–51.
20. Sim R, Cheong DM, Wong KS, Lee BM, Liew QY. Prospective randomized, double-blind, placebo-controlled study of pre- and postoperative administration of a COX-2-specific inhibitor as opioid-sparing analgesia in major colorectal surgery. Colorectal Dis. 2007;9:52–60.
21. Klein M, Andersen LP, Harvald T, Rosenberg J, Goqenur I. Increased risk of anastomotic leakage with diclofenac treatment after laparoscopic colorectal surgery. Dig Surg. 2009;26:27–30.

22. Holte K, Andersen J, Jakobsen DH, Kehlet H. Cyclo-oxygenase 2 inhibitors and the risk of anastomotic leakage after fast track colonic surgery. Br J Surg. 2009;96:650–4.
23. White PF. Changing the role of COX-2 inhibitors in the perioperative period: is paracoxib really the answer? Anesth Analg. 2005;100:1306–8.
24. Mallet C, Daulhac L, Bonnefort J, Ledent C, Etienne M, Chapuy E, et al. Endocannabinoid and serotonergic systems are needed for acetaminophen-induced analgesia. J Pain. 2008;139: 190–200.
25. White PF, Kehlet H, Neal JM, Schricker T, Carr DB. The role of the anesthesiologist in fast-track surgery: from multimodal analgesia to perioperative medical care. Anesth Analg. 2007;104:1380–96.
26. Ong CKS, Seymour RA, Lirk P, Merry AF. Combining paracetamol (acetaminophen) with Nonsteroidal Antinflammatory drugs: a qualitative systematic review of analgesic efficacy for acute postoperative pain. Anaesth Analg. 2010;110:1170–9.
27. Marrett E, Rolin M, Beaussier M, Bonnet F. Meta-analysis of intravenous ligonocaaine and postoperative recovery after abdominal surgery. Br J Surg. 2008;95:1331–8.
28. Kaba A, Laurent SR, Detroz BJ, Sessler DI, Durieux ME, Lamy ML. Intravenous lidocaine infusion facilitates acute rehabilitation after laparoscopic cholecystectomy. Anesthesiology. 2007;106:11–8.
29. Zakine J, Samarcq D, Lorne E, Moubarak M, Montravers P, Beloucif S, et al. Postoperative ketamine administration decreases morphine consumption in major abdominal surgery: a prospective, randomized, double-blind, controlled study. Anesth Analg. 2008;106:1856–61.
30. Fawcett WJ, Haxby EJ, Male DA. Magnesium: physiology and pharmacology. Br J Anaesth. 1999;83:302–20.
31. Agarwal A, Gautam S, Agarwal S, Gupta D, Singh PK, Singh U. Evaluation of a single preoperative dose of prega balin for attenuation of postoperative pain after lap aroscopic cholecystectomy. Br J Anaesth. 2008;101:700–4.
32. Paech MJ, Goy R, Chua S, Scott K, Christmas T, Doherty DA. A randomized, placebo-controlled trial of preoperative oral pregabalin for postoperative pain relief after minor gynecological surgery. Anesth Analg. 2007;105:1449–53.
33. POISE group. Effects of extended-release metoprolol succinate in patients undergoing noncardiac surgery (POISE trial): a randomised controlled trial. Lancet. 2008;371:1839–47.

Chapter 7
Colorectal Surgery and Enhanced Recovery

Matthew G. Tutton, N. Julian H. Sturt, and Alan F. Horgan

Introduction

Enhanced recovery in colorectal cancer was first realised from the work of Kehlet's group at the Hvidovre University Hospital in Denmark in 1995 [1]. An enhanced recovery program in colorectal cancer aims to minimise the metabolic and physiological response to surgery and hence hasten recovery and subsequent hospital discharge. The potential advantages of enhanced recovery are not only pertinent to the patient and clinician but to health care systems in general, as since shorter hospital stays may lessen costs and allow the treatment of greater numbers of patients. In additional a faster return to work and productivity may benefit economies in a broader sense.

Traditional perioperative management of patients undergoing colorectal resections would start preoperatively with the institution of a low residue diet followed by full mechanical bowel preparation and a prolonged period of starvation. Operations would be performed using long mid-line or paramedian incisions crossing multiple dermatomes. Postoperatively patients would often have nasogastric tubes left in situ for a number of days. Large volumes of intravenous fluids would be given and urinary catheters left in place for prolonged periods. Patients were allowed no or little oral intake in the first few days after surgery with only a gradual

M.G. Tutton (✉)
ICENI unit, General Surgery, Colchester Hospital University NHS Foundation Trust,
Colchester, Essex, UK
e-mail: matthew.tutton@colchesterhospital.nhs.uk

N.J.H. Sturt
Department of Surgery, Southend University Hospital NHS Trust, Westcliff-on-Sea, Essex, UK

A.F. Horgan
Department of Surgery, Freeman Hospital, Newcastle, UK

N. Francis et al. (eds.), *Manual of Fast Track Recovery for Colorectal Surgery*,
Enhanced Recovery, DOI 10.1007/978-0-85729-953-6_7,
© Springer-Verlag London Limited 2012

reintroduction starting with sips of water and slowly building up to diet. Sometimes this gradual reintroduction would only be commenced after the patient's bowels had worked. Analgesia was often suboptimal with subsequent limitation to patients' mobility and respiratory function. The net result of such management was often an exaggerated physiological response to trauma.

The concept of enhanced recovery for bowel surgery aims to decrease this metabolic response to trauma, hasten return to normal bowel function, facilitate early discharge from hospital and return to normal activities. As described in earlier chapters, the key elements of an enhanced recovery programme start preoperatively with adequate patient education from both colorectal specialist nurses and where appropriate stoma nurses. Mechanical bowel preparation and prolonged preoperative starving are avoided and carbohydrate loading is administered. Intraoperatively, transverse incisions or laparoscopic incisions are used; epidural analgesia and careful intraoperative fluid management are necessary. Postoperatively opioid analgesics are avoided, early and supplemented nutrition is encouraged and aggressive mobilisation and rehabilitation commenced.

This chapter focuses on the surgical techniques aimed to facilitate an enhanced recovery in colorectal surgery, explores any advantage of laparoscopic surgery and suggests how to treat complications that may arise during the patient's recovery.

Components of an Enhanced Recovery Programme in Colorectal Surgery

The individual importance of separate components of an enhanced recovery programme is difficult to evaluate and different studies have selected various elements. Kehlet et al. and the ERAS study group proposed 15 components and Wind [2] summarised 17 key elements in a systematic review (Table 7.1). There is no consensus as to the importance of the individual elements of an enhanced recovery programme and which elements are essential to clinical care in an enhanced recovery programme. Comparison between studies is difficult and different protocols 'pick and choose' different elements from a range of components. As a result of the large number of elements contained in many enhanced recovery programs it is difficult to determine which may be omitted without having a detrimental effect on the whole program. Table 7.2 outlines an established enhanced recovery programme. This chapter focuses on components that are more specific to colorectal surgery.

No Mechanical Bowel Preparation

Mechanical bowel preparation for colorectal resections has been one of the traditional surgical dogmas. The rationale for mechanical bowel preparation is based on the belief that this has a protective effect against the consequences of anastomotic

Table 7.1 Components of an enhanced recovery program

	Enhanced recovery	Rationale
1	Preoperative education and stoma training	Patient education, outlining the program and components and expectations for discharge
2	Carbohydrate loading preoperatively and avoidance of prolonged starving	Avoidance of insulin resistance
3	Use of preoperative probiotics	Induce favourable gut flora
4	No mechanical bowel preparation	Avoidance of dehydration and fluid shifts
5	No pre-medication	Minimise effects of anaesthesia
6	Goal-directed perioperative fluid administration	Avoidance of fluid overload
7	High perioperative O_2 concentrations	Maximise O_2 delivery to tissues
8	Maintenance of normothermia	Avoid deleterious effects of hypothermia on body physiology
9	Epidural analgesia	Excellent pain control and minimise affects of surgery on respiratory function
10	Laparoscopic surgery or transverse incisions	Less postoperative pain and tissue trauma
11	Avoidance of nasogastric tubes	Promote gut function
12	Avoidance of drains	Avoid effects on mobilisation and less pain
13	Avoidance of opioid analgesia	Avoidance of postoperative ileus
14	Use of postoperative laxatives	Encourage bowel function
15	Early removal of bladder catheter	Encourage mobilisation, allow early discharge
16	Enforced early mobilisation	Favourable effects on respiratory function
17	Enforced early postoperative oral feeding	Beneficial effects on gut recovery and function

leakage and infectious complications. There is now however a range of randomised trials [3–11], systemic reviews and meta-analyses [12–17] that support the avoidance of mechanical bowel preparation. Overall these have shown that there is no difference in terms of surgical outcome in terms of anastomotic leakage, mortality rates, infectious outcomes and need for re-operation between patients who have mechanical bowel preparation for colorectal surgery and those who do not. Furthermore, as well as being an unpleasant experience, in subgroups of patients such as those with renal dysfunction and elderly patients, mechanical bowel preparation can result in serious complications. These include large fluid shifts, dehydration and hypotension under anaesthesia, electrolyte disturbance, acute renal failure and in one meta-analysis a higher incidence of postoperative cardiac events [13].

Stoma Training

Additional time, education and preoperative counselling for patients who will require a stoma is required. The stoma nurse plays an essential role from the initial diagnosis, through treatment and recovery in hospital and at home [18,19]. The introduction of dummy packs preoperatively enables the patient to become familiar with the concept of a stoma and to practice positioning and changing stoma bags.

Table 7.2 Example of an enhanced recovery program in colorectal surgery (Colchester Hospital University NHS Foundation Trust)

Day before/after surgery	Protocol
1 week before	Pre-assessment visit with full counselling, instructions and necessary medications given
2 days before	Three cartons of Fresubin® (nutritional supplement) through the day
	Two sennakot (laxative) tablets in evening (left-sided resections only)
1 day before	Low-residue diet
	Three cartons of Fresubin® through day
	50 mL Infacol® (Simethicone 40 mg/mL) liquid orally in evening
	40 mg Clexane® (enoxaparin) s.c. as thromboprophylaxis at 6 pm
	One can of Maxijul® (carbohydrate) drink at 8 pm
	One can of Maxijul® drink at 10 pm
Day of surgery	One can of Maxijul® at 7 am
	Admission to hospital
	Thrombo-embolic deterrent stockings
	Phosphate enema at 7 am (left-sided resections only)
	Admission to operating theatre
	Epidural sited
	Urinary catheter sited
	Laparoscopic operation
	Minimal perioperative i.v. fluid
	Active perioperative warming with Bair Hugger®
	No nasogastric drainage
	Abdominal drains only for surgery within the pelvis
	Drink in recovery ward
	Epidural analgesia supplemented with paracetamol 1 g qds
	Rescue opiate analgesia
	Minimal postoperative i.v. fluids
	Diet started in evening
	40 mg clexane s.c. at 6 pm
Postoperative day 1	Three cartons of Fresubin® throughout day
	Normal diet as tolerated
	Abdominal drain removed (if present)
	Epidural analgesia supplemented with paracetamol 1 g qds
	Rescue opiate analgesia
	Enforced mobilisation
	i.v. fluids discontinued if patient drinking adequately
	40 mg clexane® s.c. at 6 pm
Postoperative day 2	Urinary catheter removed (except men with prostastic symptoms)
	Three cartons of Fresubin® throughout day
	Normal diet as tolerated
	Epidural analgesia supplemented with paracetamol 1 g qds
	Rescue opiate analgesia
	Enforced mobilisation
	40 mg clexane® s.c. at 6 pm
Postoperative day 3	Epidural infusion stopped at 6 am
	Urinary catheter removed (men with prostatic symptoms)

Table 7.2 (continued)

Day before/after surgery	Protocol
	Epidural catheter removed by 12 mid-day if pain is well controlled with oral analgesia
	1 paracetamol qds with rescue opiate analgesia
	Three cartons of Fresubin® throughout day
	Normal diet as tolerated
	Enforced mobilisation
	40 mg clexane® s.c. at 6 pm
Postoperative day 4	Aim for discharge home
	Paracetamol analgesia with opiate rescue
	Laxatives if necessary
	Thrombo-embolic deterrent stockings to be worn for 2 weeks
	Direct cell phone number of Nurse Practitioner (or on-call Surgical Registrar) given for patient to contact if any problems at home

This will provide an opportunity to allay fears and to improve management postoperatively. It has been shown that intensive preoperative education of patients with regard to stoma management using a combination of DVDs, mannequins and templates over two sessions can result in the achievement of stoma competency before surgery and reduce postoperative hospital stay significantly.

Preoperative carbohydrate administration involves the administration of a Maltodextran drink to patients the night before (100 g) and the morning of surgery (50 g 2 h preoperatively). Whilst studies are small, there is evidence that this will promote the feeling of well-being in patients by avoiding the period of prolonged fast preoperatively. It has also been shown to reduce the insulin resistance that is experienced following major operative procedures and to lead to a reduction of length of hospital stay.

Goal-Directed Perioperative Fluid Administration

Individualised goal-directed therapy aims to avoid perioperative hypovolaemia or fluid overload by the maximisation of flow-related haemodynamic parameters. By optimising haemodynamic and oxygen transport goals during the perioperative period this aims to prevent organ dysfunction, reduce postoperative morbidity, reduce unplanned admissions to intensive care facilities and shorten hospital stay [20]. This may even improve long-term outcome in selected patients [21]. Inadequate fluid replacement can result in organ hypoperfusion, organ dysfunction and bacterial translocation from the GI tract resulting in sepsis. Excessive fluid overload compromises cardiac function and delays the onset of gut function. Intraoperative fluid replacement can be accurately guided by the use of an oesophageal Doppler probe against indicators of cardiac output [22]. This can be very important during laparoscopic colorectal surgery as a result of the change in haemodynamic parameters both from the pneumoperitoneum and also extremes of tilt in patient positioning.

Improvements in outcomes in colorectal surgery have been reported in both open and laparoscopic series [23, 24] with studies showing reduced hospital stay, reduced complications and earlier return to gut function with goal-directed therapy in comparison to conventional intraoperative fluid replacement [25].

High Perioperative O_2 Concentrations

High perioperative oxygen concentrations aim to increase the tissue oxygen tension in the surgical wound and in colorectal anastomoses. A higher tissue oxygen tension may improve tissue healing, inducing collagen formation, neovascularisation and oxidative killing by neutrophils [26, 27]. The outcome of clinical trials in surgical patients however has shown some variable results. However, the majority of studies report a reduction in the incidence of surgical wound infections in those given perioperative-inspired oxygen at 80% when compared to more standard management with inspired oxygen concentrations around the 30% mark [28–30]; one study has reported a potential deleterious action with a higher wound infection rate [31] and others no benefit [32].

Maintenance of Normothermia

Normothermia relates to maintaining a normal adult temperature between 36.5°C and 37.5°C. Patients undergoing colorectal surgery are at risk of developing hypothermia along their surgical pathway. During anaesthesia, core temperature can drop to 35°C within the first half-hour of the procedure. This results from exposure of the patient during the procedure along with impairment of thermoregulatory mechanisms under general anaesthesia, and anaesthesia-induced peripheral vasodilatation. To prevent this, the patient's temperature should be monitored closely during surgery, fluid and blood should be warmed with a warming device to 37°C and forced air warming devices should be utilised. These practices should continue in the recovery room to ensure that on return to the ward the patient is normothermic.

Consequences of hypothermia include altered immune response and may result in an increase in surgical site infections by triggering thermoregulatory vasoconstriction with a resultant reduction in tissue oxygen tension [33]. Warming is important in patients undergoing both open surgery with inherent temperature losses from an open abdomen, but also in laparoscopic procedures which are recognised to have a longer operating time and as such are at the same risk of hypothermia [34–36].

Epidural Analgesia

Initially epidural analgesia was a core component of an enhanced recovery programme. However, more recently with the greater use of laparoscopic surgery and other modes of analgesia such as transversus abdominis plane blocks, its routine use for all cases has been questioned.

A low thoracic epidural with fine bore catheter placed at the level of T9–T10 with a mixture of opioid and local anaesthetic results in excellent postoperative pain control. Other potential benefits of epidural analgesia include a faster resolution of any postoperative ileus from sympathetic blockade, thus allowing earlier feeding. There is also a blunted trauma-mediated neuro-endocrine stress response with reduced cortisol and catecholamine release [37–41], although this has not translated into a shorter hospital stay. The potential disadvantages of epidural analgesia include urinary retention, which may result in delayed catheter removal hindering mobilisation, and postoperative hypotension due to vasodilatation, which may be difficult to control simply with intravenous fluid replacement. If the epidural analgesia is to continue in these patients then a decision has to be taken with regard to the potential need for vasopressor support [42]. Worries regarding whether epidural analgesia may effect blood flow to a colorectal anastomosis and therefore have an influence on anastomotic healing have not been born out in more recent reviews and meta-analysis [41–45].

Comparison of epidural analgesia with patient-controlled analgesia has tended to show improved analgesia with the epidural delivery of opioid [41, 46–48]. Others however have reported equivalent analgesic results with a multimodal regimen of opioid and non-steroidal analgesics with a resultant reduction in side effects such as postoperative hypotension, high-dependency stay and need for staff interventions [49].

The role of epidural analgesia in laparoscopic colorectal resections has been debated; pain requirements tend to be reduced as a result of the less invasive nature of the surgery and the smaller incisions used. However, some authors have reported earlier return of normal gut function and eating and as such shorter hospital stays with routine use [40]. More recently the use of transversus abdominis blocks has been explored and there is evidence that these reduce postoperative analgesia requirement with minimal risk and avoid the rare but serious potential complications of epidural analgesia [50–52]. Similarly the use of intrathecal analgesia has been shown to have some advantages over epidural analgesia for patients undergoing laparoscopic colorectal surgery in terms of reduced postoperative pain scores, earlier return to mobility and shorter hospital stay.

Patient Positioning

During laparoscopic procedures extreme tilt is often used throughout the procedure. For left-sided and rectal resections, extremes of head down position are frequently used to allow positioning of the small bowel and adequate intra-abdominal views of the operative field. This can have pronounced influences on cardiopulmonary function as well as cerebral blood flow. To aid postoperative recovery, prolonged use of such positions can result in both cerebral and occipital oedema and extremes of tilt should be kept to a minimum as exposure of the operative field allows. Similarly, abdominal insufflation pressures should be kept as low as will allow adequate distension of the abdomen as higher pressures are also recognised to have a deleterious effect on cardiopulmonary function as well as contributing to increased postoperative pain [53, 54].

Prolonged use of the lithotomy position has been recognised as a cause for postoperative compartment syndrome, which can result in neurovascular damage and permanent disability [55]. The addition of steep head down tilt to the patient already in the lithotomy position increases the risk of postoperative compartment syndrome and should therefore be avoided for long duration without periods of rest with restoration of blood flow to the lower extremities [56].

Laparoscopic Surgery or Transverse Incisions

Avoiding unnecessary trauma and insult is a fundamental principle of an enhanced recovery programme. By its very nature laparoscopic surgery reduces the extent of surgical trauma with minimally invasive techniques reducing surgical incisions to a minimum. This is also achieved with no detriment in the quality of surgery with longer-term oncological outcomes from laparoscopic colorectal cancer surgery demonstrating at least equivalent results when compared to open colorectal cancer surgery [57–63]. Studies that compare laparoscopic versus conventional open colorectal surgery show a reduced stay in the laparoscopic cohort compared to the open group, usually of a couple of days [64, 65]. Although there is not extensive prospectively randomised data comparing laparoscopic surgery with conventional surgery in an enhanced recovery programme, studies have shown that the advantages of laparoscopic surgery are maintained compared to conventional surgery with some suggesting a survival advantage and lower readmission rate over conventional surgery [66–69]. At present there are two multi-center prospective randomised trials that aim to strengthen the current evidence within the literature (the LAFA trial – laparoscopic and/or fast track multi-modal management and the EnRoL trial – conventional versus laparoscopic surgery for colorectal cancer within an enhanced recovery programme) [70].

It should also be noted that the enhanced recovery from laparoscopic surgery results in a quicker discharge from hospital with a faster return to normal activities, a quicker return to feeling subjectively fully recovered and resumption of activities such as driving [66, 71]. It is also possible that in the longer term the incidence of other morbidities will be reduced including adhesive intestinal obstruction and incisional herniation [60].

In institutions where laparoscopic surgery is not feasible then, where possible, there is good evidence that a transverse incision results in less pain and postoperative analgesic requirement compared with a mid-line incision [72–76].

In the case of difficult pelvic surgery it is possible to combine the concept of laparoscopic surgery and transverse incisions by means of mobilising the splenic flexure and division of the vascular structures laparoscopically followed by the performance of the rectal surgery through a low transverse incision.

Avoidance of Nasogastric Tubes

Nasogastric tubes have traditionally been employed after colorectal surgery. Their use is intended to hasten gastric emptying, prevent aspiration and pulmonary complications and diminish the risk of anastomotic leakage. Historically nasogastric tubes were left in situ until passage of flatus or faeces. With introduction of laparoscopic techniques and less invasive surgery and reduced ileus with a subsequent faster return to normal diet the avoidance of nasogastric tubes has been extended to both laparoscopic resections and open surgery [77]. Evidence also shows that their use has slowly been reducing [78]. Moreover a Cochrane meta-analysis has reported that routine nasogastric use actually increases the risk of the complications that they aim to reduce, namely longer duration of ileus and higher pulmonary complications with no protective action on a colorectal anastomosis [79].

Avoidance of Drains

Routine drainage of colorectal anastomosis, in particular rectal, has been conventional practice with the aim to drain any collection or anastomotic leakage. However, drains result in discomfort and are a hindrance to early mobilisation. Although there is some debate in the literature as to whether drain fluid can lead to earlier detection of an anastomotic leak or reduce the need for re-operation by draining the resulting pelvic collection [80], there are multiple studies and meta-analyses that have shown no advantage to routine abdominal or pelvic drainage for colorectal surgery in terms of both morbidity and mortality [81–86].

Use of Postoperative Laxatives

Laxatives can be used to encourage earlier return of bowel function and reduce the incidence of any postoperative ileus. Both oral and per rectal preparations have been given with a resulting shortened time to passage of first stool. However this has not been shown to hasten oral intake or to shorten time to discharge [87, 88].

Early Removal of Bladder Catheter

Catheters are used routinely in colorectal resections to decompress the bladder during surgery and to allow monitoring of urine output. There has been debate regarding timing of removal of urinary catheters post-surgery especially in patients who have undergone rectal surgery or those with in-dwelling epidural catheters. The more prolonged the urinary drainage continues the higher the risk of urinary tract infections. Patients who have undergone rectal resections are reported to have a higher incidence of voiding dysfunction, however studies suggest that the majority of patients can tolerate removal of a urinary catheter on the first postoperative day [89, 90]. There have also been concerns regarding removal of urinary catheters whilst epidural analgesia is still in-situ as there is a perceived higher rate of urinary retention following removal if the epidural is still being used. A couple of studies have shown that the urinary catheter can be safely removed on the first postoperative day in the majority of patients as long as there are no specific contra-indications. Early removal is not associated with a higher rate of recatheterisation, and has also been shown to reduce the incidence of urinary tract infections and also contribute to a shorter hospital stay [91, 92].

Enhanced Recovery in Rectal Cancer

The majority of studies and reports to date have concentrated on enhanced recovery programmes in colonic resections or pooled colorectal cases. There are fewer reports of such a programme in surgery for rectal cancer [93–96] and these are selected case series or cohort studies. In open rectal cancer surgery Liu reported on 73 cases reporting a reduction in mean postoperative stay of 4 days associated with a significantly reduced complication rate [94]. Delaney's group have reported a small series with a very short mean hospital stay in patients undergoing a standardised laparoscopic resection within an enhanced recovery programme. Thirty-seven patients had a mean stay of 3 days with 90% being discharged within 5 days, with a very low complication rate of 8% and no anastomotic leaks [95]. Branagan in a retrospective cohort comparison reported reduction in in-patient stays of 4 days, both in patients undergoing rectal surgery either by an open or laparoscopic route [96]. However, Chen has cautioned that there was a higher failure in completion of an enhanced recovery programme in patients with low rectal lesions [97]. Taking these preliminary studies it would appear that a similar return to normal functioning after rectal surgery with a concurrent reduction in hospital stay is possible within an enhanced recovery programme for rectal surgery as with colonic surgery. Although most studies have found rectal resections tend to have a longer in-patient stay than colonic surgery, Delaney's group achieved mean hospital stays in a selected cohort similar to the shortest reported for colonic surgery.

Single-Port Surgery

More recently the use of single-incision laparoscopic surgery (SILS) or laparoendoscopic single-site surgery (LESS) has been used in selected colorectal resections. To date there is only a limited number of cases and reports in the literature describing early experiences with the use of SILS [98–101]. The aim of single-port surgery is to reduce the surgical trauma further, limiting trauma to the abdominal wall and reducing the transparietal ports to just one from the three to six commonly employed during laparoscopic colorectal surgery. There are now reports of all common complex colorectal resections being performed entirely through a single umbilical incision or chosen stoma site. Some small series also report patient recovery in terms of hours rather than days and this has caused some authors to question whether a multimodal enhanced recovery programme after large bowel resection using single-port surgery is even necessary with single-port surgery [99, 101, 102]. However, the techniques required for single-port surgery are still being developed and randomised controlled trials comparing single-port surgery to laparoscopic surgery within enhanced recovery programmes are required.

Benefits of Enhanced Recovery Programme

There are now a number of meta-analyses that have examined the reported benefits of an enhanced recovery programme. Given the different methodologies applied and potential components as described above there are obvious variation in results. The predominant end points that have been analysed include short-term morbidity, length of postoperative stay, re-admission rates and mortality. Meta-analyses of randomised trials of more than 1,000 patients now show that both the length of hospital stay and complication and morbidity rates are significantly reduced in an enhanced recovery group when compared to conventional surgery. No significant difference has been shown in terms of re-admission rates or in mortality [2, 103–106]. Although individual series and studies suggest an additional benefit of laparoscopic surgery within an enhanced recovery programme, the results of larger randomised trials are awaited before definitive conclusions can be drawn [104, 107, 108].

Recognising Complications Within an Enhanced Recovery Programme

As with any operation patients recovering from colorectal resections within an enhanced recovery programme are at risk of complications. Recognition is important as the earlier the intervention the more likely it will result in a quick and beneficial outcome [109]. Common complications include nausea and vomiting, postoperative ileus, failure to mobilise and also less commonly postoperative haemorrhage, anastomotic leak or intra-abdominal collections.

Nausea and Vomiting

Nausea and/or vomiting are common in all postoperative surgical patients. Anaesthetic considerations that help reduce postoperative nausea and vomiting include avoiding nitrous oxide and volatile inhaled anaesthetic agents as well as providing supplemental oxygen. However, an enhanced recovery programme aims to encourage oral intake within the first few hours of recovery from anaesthesia. A proportion of patients will find this difficult to tolerate and a regular anti-emetic is often enough to allow an adequate oral intake to be commenced. A wide variety of anti-emetics with differing mechanisms of action are available to manage postoperative nausea. A low-dose 5-HT$_3$ receptor antagonist is often used as first-line management. If this fails, then addition of dexamethasone or a dopamine antagonist would be a suitable second line approach. Use of any other rescue anti-emetic should then be from a differing drug class [110]. If vomiting fails to settle or there are other signs such as distension, increased pain or tachycardia then other complications should be considered.

Postoperative Ileus

A postoperative ileus following surgery is a common cause for vomiting that fails to settle. It has been defined as delay in gastrointestinal motility beyond 3 days [111]. A significant component of an enhanced recovery programme is seeking to avoid factors that are known to contribute to a postoperative ileus. As noted previously, the type of anaesthetic, goal-directed therapy, avoiding over-hydration and electrolyte disturbance, limited use of opioid analgesia and early mobilisation all aim to minimise the risk of postoperative ileus.

However, once ileus is established then oral intake should cease. Exclusion of other causes for an ileus such as anastomotic leakage or an intra-abdominal collection should be considered as well as exclusion of a mechanical obstruction. CT scanning is the modality of choice if any diagnostic doubt exists. Treatment then includes the passage of a nasogastric tube to decompress the stomach and support of hydration with intravenous fluids. Careful fluid balance is maintained to prevent either dehydration or over-hydration and any related electrolyte disturbance is corrected. If the ileus is prolonged beyond 7 days postoperatively then parenteral nutrition should be considered [112]. Other adjunct measures that have been used to shorten ileus with some reported success include chewing gum, which stimulates bowel motility [113].

Anastomotic Leak

Anastomotic leak or intra-abdominal collections are recognised complications of colorectal surgery. Although an enhanced recovery programme per se has no effect on anastomotic leak rates, anastomotic leaks will occur in approximately 3–15% of colorectal resections with the risk increasing the more distal the anastomosis [114]. Other factors known to contribute to an increased risk of anastomotic leak include preoperative use of chemoradiotherapy, inflammatory bowel disease, operative time over 200 min, blood loss of over 200 mL and a serum albumin below 35 g/L [115]. Although an extensive anastomotic leak may result in rapidly progressive signs of pyrexia, acute abdominal pain and tenderness it may be that a smaller leak or peri-anastomotic collection shows somewhat subtler signs. These may manifest signs such as a postoperative ileus, a cardiac arrythmia (commonly atrial fibrillation), a tachycardia with pyrexia, or simply slow recovery and failure to progress. In these cases a high index of suspicion is needed and appropriate investigation with either contrast-enhanced CT scanning or a water-soluble contrast enema be performed early. Even if CT scanning is reassuring if the clinical condition deteriorates then a diagnostic laparoscopy, particularly in patients who have had laparoscopic resections, is a rapid means of achieving a diagnosis and examining the integrity of the anastomosis. Treatment options will depend on the clinical state and extent of any leak or collection and will range from percutaneous drainage, laparoscopic irrigation and drainage, defunctioning stomas or Hartmann's procedure to more extensive laparotomy or laparostomy in the most severe cases of faecal peritonitis.

One frequently expressed concern is with a shorter length of stay is whether an anastomotic leak will present after discharge from hospital at home with disastrous consequences. In the authors' experience, within an enhanced recovery programme, the faster return of normal gastrointestinal function results in the signs of an anastomotic leak becoming apparent at an earlier stage than classically quoted and usually present on the second to third postoperative day. In the vast majority of patients, complications are identified long before plans for discharge are made. As part of continued care once discharged home, instructions are given to make immediate contact with one of the enhanced recovery nurses if the patient has any concerns.

Conclusions

There is now extensive evidence that enhanced recovery programmes benefit the recovery of colorectal patients, clinicians and health care systems. A well-run programme reduces the physiological response to the tissue insult from surgery and as a result there is less postoperative pain, fewer complications, a shorter hospital stay and faster recovery and return to work. Although the case for laparoscopic surgery remains to be proven explicitly, the attendant advantages that minimal access surgery brings and the reduced tissue trauma inherent to this approach would seem to make it an ideal partner for an enhanced recovery programme in colorectal surgery.

References

1. Bardram L, Funch-Jensen P, Jensen P, Crawford ME, Kehlet H. Recovery after laparoscopic colonic surgery with epidural analgesia, and early oral nutrition and mobilisation. Lancet. 1995;345(8952):763–4.

2. Wind J, Polle SW, Fung Kon Jin PH, Dejong CH, von Meyenfeldt MF, Ubbink DT, et al. Systematic review of enhanced recovery programmes in colonic surgery. Br J Surg. 2006;93(7): 800–9.

3. Burke P, Mealy K, Gillen P, Joyce W, Traynor O, Hyland J. Requirement for bowel preparation in colorectal surgery. Br J Surg. 1994;81(6):907–10.

4. Miettinen RP, Laitinen ST, Makela JT, Paakkonen ME. Bowel preparation with oral polyethylene glycol electrolyte solution vs. no preparation in elective open colorectal surgery: prospective, randomized study. Dis Colon Rectum. 2000;43(5):669–75; discussion 75–7.

5. Santos Jr JC, Batista J, Sirimarco MT, Guimaraes AS, Levy CE. Prospective randomized trial of mechanical bowel preparation in patients undergoing elective colorectal surgery. Br J Surg. 1994;81(11):1673–6.

6. Bucher P, Gervaz P, Soravia C, Mermillod B, Erne M, Morel P. Randomized clinical trial of mechanical bowel preparation versus no preparation before elective left-sided colorectal surgery. Br J Surg. 2005;92(4):409–14.

7. Contant CM, Hop WC, Van't Sant HP, Oostvogel HJ, Smeets HJ, Stassen LP, et al. Mechanical bowel preparation for elective colorectal surgery: a multicentre randomised trial. Lancet. 2007;370(9605):2112–7.

8. Fa-Si-Oen P, Roumen R, Buitenweg J, van de Velde C, van Geldere D, Putter H, et al. Mechanical bowel preparation or not? Outcome of a multicenter, randomized trial in elective open colon surgery. Dis Colon Rectum. 2005;48(8):1509–616.

9. Pena-Soria MJ, Mayol JM, Anula-Fernandez R, Arbeo-Escolar A, Fernandez-Represa JA. Mechanical bowel preparation for elective colorectal surgery with primary intraperitoneal anastomosis by a single surgeon: interim analysis of a prospective single-blinded randomized trial. J Gastrointest Surg. 2007;11(5):562–7.

10. Ram E, Sherman Y, Weil R, Vishne T, Kravarusic D, Dreznik Z. Is mechanical bowel preparation mandatory for elective colon surgery? A prospective randomized study. Arch Surg. 2005;140(3):285–8.

11. Zmora O, Mahajna A, Bar-Zakai B, Rosin D, Hershko D, Shabtai M, et al. Colon and rectal surgery without mechanical bowel preparation: a randomized prospective trial. Ann Surg. 2003;237(3):363–7.

12. Bucher P, Mermillod B, Gervaz P, Morel P. Mechanical bowel preparation for elective colorectal surgery: a meta-analysis. Arch Surg. 2004;139(12):1359–64; discussion 65.

13. Gravante G, Caruso R, Andreani SM, Giordano P. Mechanical bowel preparation for colorectal surgery: a meta-analysis on abdominal and systemic complications on almost 5,000 patients. Int J Colorectal Dis. 2008;23(12):1145–50.

14. Pineda CE, Shelton AA, Hernandez-Boussard T, Morton JM, Welton ML. Mechanical bowel preparation in intestinal surgery: a meta-analysis and review of the literature. J Gastrointest Surg. 2008;12(11):2037–44.

15. Slim K, Vicaut E, Launay-Savary MV, Contant C, Chipponi J. Updated systematic review and meta-analysis of randomized clinical trials on the role of mechanical bowel preparation before colorectal surgery. Ann Surg. 2009;249(2):203–9.

16. Wille-Jorgensen P, Guenaga KF, Matos D, Castro AA. Pre-operative mechanical bowel cleansing or not? an updated meta-analysis. Colorectal Dis. 2005;7(4):304–10.

17. Guenaga KK, Matos D, Wille-Jorgensen P. Mechanical bowel preparation for elective colorectal surgery. Cochrane Database Syst Rev. 2009;(1):CD001544.

18. Comb J. Role of the stoma care nurse: patients with cancer and colostomy. Br J Nurs. 2003;12(14):852–6.

19. Lee J. Nurse prescribing in practice: patient choice in stoma care. Br J Community Nurs. 2001;6(1):33–7.

20. Lees N, Hamilton M, Rhodes A. Clinical review: goal-directed therapy in high risk surgical patients. Crit Care. 2009;13(5):231.

21. Rhodes A, Cecconi M, Hamilton M, Poloniecki J, Woods J, Boyd O, et al. Goal-directed therapy in high-risk surgical patients: a 15-year follow-up study. Intensive Care Med. 2010;36(8):1327–32. Epub 2010 Apr 8.

22. Noblett SE, Snowden CP, Shenton BK, Horgan AF. Randomized clinical trial assessing the effect of Doppler-optimized fluid management on outcome after elective colorectal resection. Br J Surg. 2006;93(9):1069–76.
23. Senagore AJ, Emery T, Luchtefeld M, Kim D, Dujovny N, Hoedema R. Fluid management for laparoscopic colectomy: a prospective, randomized assessment of goal-directed administration of balanced salt solution or hetastarch coupled with an enhanced recovery program. Dis Colon Rectum. 2009;52(12):1935–40.
24. Gan TJ, Soppitt A, Maroof M, el-Moalem H, Robertson KM, Moretti E, et al. Goal-directed intraoperative fluid administration reduces length of hospital stay after major surgery. Anesthesiology. 2002;97(4):820–6.
25. Bundgaard-Nielsen M, Holte K, Secher NH, Kehlet H. Monitoring of peri-operative fluid administration by individualized goal-directed therapy. Acta Anaesthesiol Scand. 2007;51(3): 331–40.
26. Allen DB, Maguire JJ, Mahdavian M, Wicke C, Marcocci L, Scheuenstuhl H, et al. Wound hypoxia and acidosis limit neutrophil bacterial killing mechanisms. Arch Surg. 1997;132(9):991–6.
27. Hopf HW, Holm J. Hyperoxia and infection. Best Pract Res Clin Anaesthesiol. 2008;22(3): 553–69.
28. Belda FJ, Aguilera L, Garcia de la Asuncion J, Alberti J, Vicente R, Ferrandiz L, et al. Supplemental perioperative oxygen and the risk of surgical wound infection: a randomized controlled trial. JAMA. 2005;294(16):2035–42.
29. Brasel K, McRitchie D, Dellinger P. Canadian Association of General Surgeons and American College of Surgeons Evidence Based Reviews in Surgery. 21: the risk of surgical site infection is reduced with perioperative oxygen. Can J Surg. 2007;50(3):214–6.
30. Greif R, Akca O, Horn EP, Kurz A, Sessler DI. Supplemental perioperative oxygen to reduce the incidence of surgical-wound infection. Outcomes Research Group. N Engl J Med. 2000;342(3):161–7.
31. Pryor KO, Fahey 3rd TJ, Lien CA, Goldstein PA. Surgical site infection and the routine use of perioperative hyperoxia in a general surgical population: a randomized controlled trial. JAMA. 2004;291(1):79–87.
32. Meyhoff CS, Wetterslev J, Jorgensen LN, Henneberg SW, Hogdall C, Lundvall L, et al. Effect of high perioperative oxygen fraction on surgical site infection and pulmonary complications after abdominal surgery: the PROXI randomized clinical trial. JAMA. 2009;302(14):1543–50.
33. Kurz A, Sessler DI, Lenhardt R. Perioperative normothermia to reduce the incidence of surgical-wound infection and shorten hospitalization. Study of Wound Infection and Temperature Group. N Engl J Med. 1996;334(19):1209–515.
34. Luck AJ, Moyes D, Maddern GJ, Hewett PJ. Core temperature changes during open and laparoscopic colorectal surgery. Surg Endosc. 1999;13(5):480–3.
35. Danelli G, Berti M, Perotti V, Albertin A, Baccari P, Deni F, et al. Temperature control and recovery of bowel function after laparoscopic or laparotomic colorectal surgery in patients receiving combined epidural/general anesthesia and postoperative epidural analgesia. Anesth Analg. 2002;95(2):467–71, table of contents.
36. Stewart BT, Stitz RW, Tuch MM, Lumley JW. Hypothermia in open and laparoscopic colorectal surgery. Dis Colon Rectum. 1999;42(10):1292–5.
37. Senagore AJ, Whalley D, Delaney CP, Mekhail N, Duepree HJ, Fazio VW. Epidural anesthesia-analgesia shortens length of stay after laparoscopic segmental colectomy for benign pathology. Surgery. 2001;129(6):672–6.
38. Neudecker J, Schwenk W, Junghans T, Pietsch S, Bohm B, Muller JM. Randomized controlled trial to examine the influence of thoracic epidural analgesia on postoperative ileus after laparoscopic sigmoid resection. Br J Surg. 1999;86(10):1292–5.
39. Malenkovic V, Baricevic I, Jones DR, Nedic O, Bilanovic D. Enhanced suppression of hormonal and metabolic responses to stress by application of combined spinal-epidural and general anaesthesia compared with combined spinal general anaesthesia during colorectal surgery. Chirurgia (Bucur). 2008;103(2):205–10.

40. Taqi A, Hong X, Mistraletti G, Stein B, Charlebois P, Carli F. Thoracic epidural analgesia facilitates the restoration of bowel function and dietary intake in patients undergoing laparoscopic colon resection using a traditional, nonaccelerated, perioperative care program. Surg Endosc. 2007;21(2):247–52.

41. Carlstedt A, Nordgren S, Fasth S, Appelgren L, Hulten L. Epidural anaesthesia and postoperative colorectal motility–a possible hazard to a colorectal anastomosis. Int J Colorectal Dis. 1989;4(3):144–9.

42. Marret E, Remy C, Bonnet F. Meta-analysis of epidural analgesia versus parenteral opioid analgesia after colorectal surgery. Br J Surg. 2007;94(6):665–73.

43. Sala C, Garcia-Granero E, Molina MJ, Garcia JV, Lledo S. Effect of epidural anesthesia on colorectal anastomosis: a tonometric assessment. Dis Colon Rectum. 1997;40(8):958–61.

44. Schnitzler M, Kilbride MJ, Senagore A. Effect of epidural analgesia on colorectal anastomotic healing and colonic motility. Reg Anesth. 1992;17(3):143–7.

45. Rimaitis K, Pavalkis D. Does epidural anaesthesia and analgesia really improves surgical outcome after colorectal cancer surgery? Acta Chir Iugosl. 2006;53(2):85–9.

46. Turunen P, Carpelan-Holmstrom M, Kairaluoma P, Wikstrom H, Kruuna O, Pere P, et al. Epidural analgesia diminished pain but did not otherwise improve enhanced recovery after laparoscopic sigmoidectomy: a prospective randomized study. Surg Endosc. 2009;23(1):31–7.

47. Gendall KA, Kennedy RR, Watson AJ, Frizelle FA. The effect of epidural analgesia on postoperative outcome after colorectal surgery. Colorectal Dis. 2007;9(7):584–98; discussion 98–600.

48. Beaussier M, Weickmans H, Parc Y, Delpierre E, Camus Y, Funck-Brentano C, et al. Postoperative analgesia and recovery course after major colorectal surgery in elderly patients: a randomized comparison between intrathecal morphine and intravenous PCA morphine. Reg Anesth Pain Med. 2006;31(6):531–8.

49. Chilvers CR, Nguyen MH, Robertson IK. Changing from epidural to multimodal analgesia for colorectal laparotomy: an audit. Anaesth Intensive Care. 2007;35(2):230–8.

50. Conaghan P, Maxwell-Armstrong C, Bedforth N, Gornall C, Baxendale B, Hong LL, et al. Efficacy of transversus abdominis plane blocks in laparoscopic colorectal resections. Surg Endosc. 2010;24(10):2480–4. Epub 2010 Apr 8.

51. Zingg U, Miskovic D, Hamel CT, Erni L, Oertli D, Metzger U. Influence of thoracic epidural analgesia on postoperative pain relief and ileus after laparoscopic colorectal resection: benefit with epidural analgesia. Surg Endosc. 2009;23(2):276–82.

52. Zafar N, Davies R, Greenslade GL, Dixon AR. The evolution of analgesia in an "Accelerated" recovery programme for resectional laparoscopic colorectal surgery with anastomosis. Colorectal Dis. 2010;12(2):119–24.

53. Wallace DH, Serpell MG, Baxter JN, O'Dwyer PJ. Randomized trial of different insufflation pressures for laparoscopic cholecystectomy. Br J Surg. 1997;84(4):455–8.

54. Gipson CL, Johnson GA, Fisher R, Stewart A, Giles G, Johnson JO, et al. Changes in cerebral oximetry during peritoneal insufflation for laparoscopic procedures. J Minim Access Surg. 2006;2(2):67–72.

55. Frezza EE. The lithotomy versus the supine position for laparoscopic advanced surgeries: a historical review. J Laparoendosc Adv Surg Tech A. 2005;15(2):140–4.

56. Ikeya E, Taguchi J, Ohta K, Miyazaki Y, Hashimoto O, Yagi K, et al. Compartment syndrome of bilateral lower extremities following laparoscopic surgery of rectal cancer in lithotomy position: report of a case. Surg Today. 2006;36(12):1122–5.

57. Breukink S, Pierie J, Wiggers T. Laparoscopic versus open total mesorectal excision for rectal cancer. Cochrane Database Syst Rev. 2006;(4):CD005200.

58. Laurent C, Leblanc F, Wutrich P, Scheffler M, Rullier E. Laparoscopic versus open surgery for rectal cancer: long-term oncologic results. Ann Surg. 2009;250(1):54–61.

59. Buunen M, Veldkamp R, Hop WC, Kuhry E, Jeekel J, Haglind E, et al. Survival after laparoscopic surgery versus open surgery for colon cancer: long-term outcome of a randomised clinical trial. Lancet Oncol. 2009;10(1):44–52.

60. Jayne DG, Guillou PJ, Thorpe H, Quirke P, Copeland J, Smith AM, et al. Randomized trial of laparoscopic-assisted resection of colorectal carcinoma: 3-year results of the UK MRC CLASICC Trial Group. J Clin Oncol. 2007;25(21):3061–8.

61. Kuhry E, Schwenk W, Gaupset R, Romild U, Bonjer J. Long-term outcome of laparoscopic surgery for colorectal cancer: a cochrane systematic review of randomised controlled trials. Cancer Treat Rev. 2008;34(6):498–504.

62. Yamamoto S, Watanabe M, Hasegawa H, Kitajima M. Oncologic outcome of laparoscopic versus open surgery for advanced colorectal cancer. Hepatogastroenterology. 2001;48(41):1248–51.

63. Yamamoto S, Watanabe M, Hasegawa H, Baba H, Hideki N, Kitajima M. Oncologic outcome of laparoscopic surgery for T1 and T2 colorectal carcinoma. Hepatogastroenterology. 2003;50(50):396–400.

64. Braga M, Vignali A, Gianotti L, Zuliani W, Radaelli G, Gruarin P, et al. Laparoscopic versus open colorectal surgery: a randomized trial on short-term outcome. Ann Surg. 2002;236(6):759–66; discussion 67.

65. Delaney CP. Outcome of discharge within 24 to 72 hours after laparoscopic colorectal surgery. Dis Colon Rectum. 2008;51(2):181–5.

66. Raymond T, Kumar S, Dastur J, Khot U, Stewart M, et al. Case controlled study of the hospital stay and return to full activity following laparoscopic and open colorectal surgery before and after the introduction of an enhanced recovery programme. Colorectal Dis. 2010;12(10):1001–6.

67. Vlug MS, Wind J, van der Zaag E, Ubbink DT, Cense HA, Bemelman WA. Systematic review of laparoscopic vs open colonic surgery within an enhanced recovery programme. Colorectal Dis. 2009;11(4):335–43.

68. King PM, Blazeby JM, Ewings P, Franks PJ, Longman RJ, Kendrick AH, et al. Randomized clinical trial comparing laparoscopic and open surgery for colorectal cancer within an enhanced recovery programme. Br J Surg. 2006;93(3):300–8.

69. Faiz O, Brown T, Colucci G, Kennedy RH. A cohort study of results following elective colonic and rectal resection within an enhanced recovery programme. Colorectal Dis. 2009;11(4):366–72.

70. Wind J, Hofland J, Preckel B, Hollmann MW, Bossuyt PM, Gouma DJ, et al. Perioperative strategy in colonic surgery; LAparoscopy and/or FAst track multimodal management versus standard care (LAFA trial). BMC Surg. 2006;6:16.

71. King PM, Blazeby JM, Ewings P, Longman RJ, Kipling RM, Franks PJ, et al. The influence of an enhanced recovery programme on clinical outcomes, costs and quality of life after surgery for colorectal cancer. Colorectal Dis. 2006;8(6):506–13.

72. Lohsiriwat V, Lohsiriwat D, Boonnuch W, Chinswangwatanakul V, Akaraviputh T, Methasade A, et al. Comparison between midline and right transverse incision in right hemicolectomy for right-sided colon cancer: a retrospective study. J Med Assoc Thai. 2009;92(8):1003–8.

73. Lohsiriwat V, Lohsiriwat D, Chinswangwatanakul V, Akaraviputh T, Lert-Akyamanee N. Comparison of short-term outcomes between laparoscopically-assisted vs. transverse-incision open right hemicolectomy for right-sided colon cancer: a retrospective study. World J Surg Oncol. 2007;5:49.

74. Lindgren PG, Nordgren SR, Oresland T, Hulten L. Midline or transverse abdominal incision for right-sided colon cancer-a randomized trial. Colorectal Dis. 2001;3(1):46–50.

75. Trimpi HD. Transverse incision in abdominal surgery of the colon and rectum. Dis Colon Rectum. 1958;1(5):339–44.

76. Donati D, Brown SR, Eu KW, Ho YH, Seow-Choen F. Comparison between midline incision and limited right skin crease incision for right-sided colonic cancers. Tech Coloproctol. 2002;6(1):1–4.

77. Sands DR, Wexner SD. Nasogastric tubes and dietary advancement after laparoscopic and open colorectal surgery. Nutrition. 1999;15(5):347–50.

78. Roig JV, Garcia-Fadrique A, Garcia Armengol J, Villalba FL, Bruna M, Sancho C, et al. Use of nasogastric tubes and drains after colorectal surgery. Have attitudes changed in the last 10 years? Cir Esp. 2008;83(2):78–84.

79. Nelson R, Edwards S, Tse B. Prophylactic nasogastric decompression after abdominal surgery. Cochrane Database Syst Rev. 2007;(3):CD004929.
80. Tsujinaka S, Kawamura YJ, Konishi F, Maeda T, Mizokami K. Pelvic drainage for anterior resection revisited: use of drains in anastomotic leaks. ANZ J Surg. 2008;78(6):461–5.
81. Foster ME. To drain or not after colorectal surgery. Ann R Coll Surg Engl. 1988;70(3):119.
82. Fingerhut A, Msika S, Yahchouchi E, Merad F, Hay JM, Millat B. Neither pelvic nor abdominal drainage is needed after anastomosis in elective, uncomplicated, colorectal surgery. Ann Surg. 2000;231(4):613–4.
83. Merad F, Hay JM, Fingerhut A, Yahchouchi E, Laborde Y, Pelissier E, et al. Is prophylactic pelvic drainage useful after elective rectal or anal anastomosis? A multicenter controlled randomized trial. French Association for Surgical Research. Surgery. 1999;125(5):529–35.
84. Merad F, Yahchouchi E, Hay JM, Fingerhut A, Laborde Y, Langlois-Zantain O. Prophylactic abdominal drainage after elective colonic resection and suprapromontory anastomosis: a multicenter study controlled by randomization. French Associations for Surgical Research. Arch Surg. 1998;133(3):309–14.
85. Jesus EC, Karliczek A, Matos D, Castro AA, Atallah AN. Prophylactic anastomotic drainage for colorectal surgery. Cochrane Database Syst Rev. 2004;(4):CD002100.
86. Karliczek A, Jesus EC, Matos D, Castro AA, Atallah AN, Wiggers T. Drainage or nondrainage in elective colorectal anastomosis: a systematic review and meta-analysis. Colorectal Dis. 2006;8(4):259–65.
87. Wiriyakosol S, Kongdan Y, Euanorasetr C, Wacharachaisurapol N, Lertsithichai P. Randomized controlled trial of bisacodyl suppository versus placebo for postoperative ileus after elective colectomy for colon cancer. Asian J Surg. 2007;30(3):167–72.
88. Zingg U, Miskovic D, Pasternak I, Meyer P, Hamel CT, Metzger U. Effect of bisacodyl on postoperative bowel motility in elective colorectal surgery: a prospective, randomized trial. Int J Colorectal Dis. 2008;23(12):1175–83.
89. Benoist S, Panis Y, Denet C, Mauvais F, Mariani P, Valleur P. Optimal duration of urinary drainage after rectal resection: a randomized controlled trial. Surgery. 1999;125(2):135–41.
90. Zmora O, Madbouly K, Tulchinsky H, Hussein A, Khaikin M. Urinary bladder catheter drainage following pelvic surgery–is it necessary for that long? Dis Colon Rectum. 2010;53(3): 321–6.
91. Basse L, Werner M, Kehlet H. Is urinary drainage necessary during continuous epidural analgesia after colonic resection? Reg Anesth Pain Med. 2000;25(5):498–501.
92. Zaouter C, Kaneva P, Carli F. Less urinary tract infection by earlier removal of bladder catheter in surgical patients receiving thoracic epidural analgesia. Reg Anesth Pain Med. 2009;34(6): 542–8.
93. Schwenk W, Neudecker J, Raue W, Haase O, Muller JM. "Fast-track" rehabilitation after rectal cancer resection. Int J Colorectal Dis. 2006;21(6):547–53.
94. Liu Z, Wang XD, Li L. Perioperative fast track programs enhance the postoperative recovery after rectal carcinoma resection. Zhonghua Wei Chang Wai Ke Za Zhi. 2008;11(6):551–3.
95. Lindsetmo RO, Champagne B, Delaney CP. Laparoscopic rectal resections and fast-track surgery: what can be expected? Am J Surg. 2009;197(3):408–12.
96. Branagan G, Richardson L, Shetty A, Chave HS. An enhanced recovery programme reduces length of stay after rectal surgery. Int J Colorectal Dis. 2010;25(11):1359–62.
97. Chen CC, Huang IP, Liu MC, Jian JJ, Cheng SH. Is it appropriate to apply the enhanced recovery program to patients undergoing laparoscopic rectal surgery? Surg Endosc. 2011;25(5): 1477–83. Epub 2010 Oct 29.
98. Remzi FH, Kirat HT, Kaouk JH, Geisler DP. Single-port laparoscopy in colorectal surgery. Colorectal Dis. 2008;10(8):823–6.
99. Gash KJ, Goede AC, Chambers W, Greenslade GL, Dixon AR. Laparoendoscopic single-site surgery is feasible in complex colorectal resections and could enable day case colectomy. Surg Endosc. 2011;25(3):835–40.

100. Chew MH, Wong MT, Lim BY, Ng KH, Eu KW. Evaluation of current devices in single-incision laparoscopic colorectal surgery: a preliminary experience in 32 consecutive cases. World J Surg. 2011;35(4):873–80.
101. Diana M, Dhumane P, Cahill RA, Mortensen N, Leroy J, Marescaux J. Minimal invasive single-site surgery in colorectal procedures: current state of the art. J Minim Access Surg. 2011;7(1):52–60.
102. Chambers W, Bicsak M, Lamparelli M, Dixon A. Single-incision laparoscopic surgery (SILS) in complex colorectal surgery: a technique offering potential and not just cosmesis. Colorectal Dis. 2011;13(4):393–8.
103. Varadhan KK, Neal KR, Dejong CH, Fearon KC, Ljungqvist O, Lobo DN. The enhanced recovery after surgery (ERAS) pathway for patients undergoing major elective open colorectal surgery: a meta-analysis of randomized controlled trials. Clin Nutr. 2010;29(4):434–40. Epub 2010 Jan 29.
104. Eskicioglu C, Forbes SS, Aarts MA, Okrainec A, McLeod RS. Enhanced recovery after surgery (ERAS) programs for patients having colorectal surgery: a meta-analysis of randomized trials. J Gastrointest Surg. 2009;13(12):2321–9.
105. Gouvas N, Tan E, Windsor A, Xynos E, Tekkis PP. Fast-track vs standard care in colorectal surgery: a meta-analysis update. Int J Colorectal Dis. 2009;24(10):1119–31.
106. Mastracci TM, Cohen Z, Senagore A. Canadian Association of General Surgeons and American College of Surgeons Evidence-Based Reviews in Surgery. 24. Fast-track programs in colonic surgery. Systematic review of enhanced recovery programmes in colonic surgery. Can J Surg. 2008;51(1):70–2.
107. Al Chalabi H, Kavanagh DO, Hassan L, Donnell KO, Nugent E, Andrews E, et al. The benefit of an enhanced recovery programme following elective laparoscopic sigmoid colectomy. Int J Colorectal Dis. 2010;25(6):761–6. Epub 2010 Feb 23.
108. Khan S, Gatt M, MacFie J. Enhanced recovery programmes and colorectal surgery: does the laparoscope confer additional advantages? Colorectal Dis. 2009;11(9):902–8.
109. Wright S, Burch J, Jenkins JT. Enhanced recovery pathway in colorectal surgery 2: postoperative complications. Nurs Times. 2009;105(29):24–6.
110. Wilhelm SM, Dehoorne-Smith ML, Kale-Pradhan PB. Prevention of postoperative nausea and vomiting. Ann Pharmacother. 2007;41(1):68–78.
111. Bisanz A, Palmer JL, Reddy S, Cloutier L, Dixon T, Cohen MZ, et al. Characterizing postoperative paralytic ileus as evidence for future research and clinical practice. Gastroenterol Nurs. 2008;31(5):336–44.
112. Braga M, Ljungqvist O, Soeters P, Fearon K, Weimann A, Bozzetti F. ESPEN guidelines on parenteral nutrition: surgery. Clin Nutr. 2009;28(4):378–86.
113. Schuster R, Grewal N, Greaney GC, Waxman K. Gum chewing reduces ileus after elective open sigmoid colectomy. Arch Surg. 2006;141(2):174–6.
114. Matthiessen P, Hallbook O, Andersson M, Rutegard J, Sjodahl R. Risk factors for anastomotic leakage after anterior resection of the rectum. Colorectal Dis. 2004;6(6):462–9.
115. Telem DA, Chin EH, Nguyen SQ, Divino CM. Risk factors for anastomotic leak following colorectal surgery: a case-control study. Arch Surg. 2010;145(4):371–6; discussion 76.

Chapter 8
Setting Up an Enhanced Recovery Programme

Fiona Carter and Robin H. Kennedy

Introduction

The subject of this chapter is one of the most debated topics at meetings and conferences, with novice teams frequently requesting advice on how to get started with enhanced recovery (ER). The initiative usually begins through the enthusiasm of a clinical champion, who should then form a steering group of key stakeholders to oversee the introduction of ER. This group will also be responsible for the creation of a robust business case to ensure that there is appropriate management and financial backing for the venture. Creation of a new care pathway and associated literature should then follow, together with development of a suitable audit of outcomes or monitoring of the new pathway. Education of professional colleagues, patients, relatives and carers is essential to the success of the programme and it is important to begin with a pilot to test the concept. Once the new pathway has been tested and monitored, the next phase is to embed the protocols as standard practice and to refine and publicise the programme as necessary.

Discussions with expert sites, and follow-up studies with novice groups, have highlighted a number of hurdles that must be negotiated in the adoption of ER. This chapter presents some specific techniques that facilitate change management and then covers all the above issues, in addition troubleshooting and how one overcomes barriers is also reviewed.

F. Carter (✉)
Yeovil Academy, Yeovil District Hospital NHS Foundation Trust,
Yeovil, Somerset, United Kingdom

R.H. Kennedy
St. Mark's Hospital,
Harrow, United Kingdom

N. Francis et al. (eds.), *Manual of Fast Track Recovery for Colorectal Surgery*,
Enhanced Recovery, DOI 10.1007/978-0-85729-953-6_8,
© Springer-Verlag London Limited 2012

Fig. 8.1 The PDSA Cycle

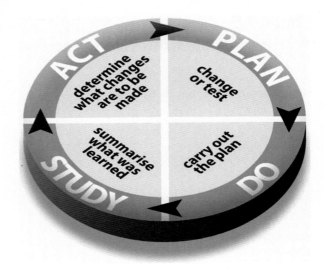

Principles of Change Management

Health care, like most other industries, resonates to the sound of the latest management technique that promises to deliver improvement. One might become cynical regarding these instructions as many people regard the introduction of change as intuitive. It is however not well done by all and it is worth reflecting on some key principles that help major transitions occur successfully and avoid missed opportunities. We look at three examples of a management techniques: the plan-do-study-act (PDSA) cycle, work published by John P. Kotter [1] on change management and the concept of 'action learning'.

The origins of the humble PDSA cycle (Fig. 8.1) originated in 1620 and are credited to Francis Bacon. The concept was popularised by Dr Edwards Deming in the mid-1900s in order to allow improvement to occur without the paralysis that may accompany change due to fears that the outcome will be wrong. Although other techniques are perhaps more in vogue now, this concept is simple to understand and useful to 'kick-start' the process of change.

John P Kotter from the Harvard Business School, spent time analysing success and failure throughout the world when companies try to make fundamental change in how they do business. He published eight key steps in a transformation strategy [1]:

1. Establishing of a sense of urgency – One might interpret this with respect to ER care as the need to grasp a major opportunity to improve patient care.
2. Forming a powerful guiding coalition – This step ensures that the group leading the change has the necessary influence and tools to achieve it.
3. Creating a vision – Can we deliver a vision that is clear and impressive enough to motivate the team who will deliver it?

4. Communicating the vision – We will touch on this later in the chapter but the important issue is that communication has to be repeated numerous times to different members/groups of staff, and often repeatedly to the same staff.
5. Empowering others to act on the vision – Solutions will come from any member of the team irrespective of their position in the 'hierarchy' and encouraging this team approach forms a powerfully motivated group. One also has to recognise that there will be certain people who might wish to impede the process of change, consciously or not, and their influence needs to be considered and dealt with appropriately.
6. Planning for and creating short-tem wins – The identification of success in the change process is important and needs to be celebrated to maintain momentum
7. Consolidating improvements and producing still more change – As success demonstrates the system is producing results, it is important to harness the momentum and complete the process.
8. Institutionalising the new approach – There may be temporary staff who guided the process of change and they, along with the new approaches, need to be permanently incorporated within the organisation to ensure leadership continues and succession occurs.

Action learning is a process developed by the physicist Reginald Revans in the 1940s. When working for the government in coal production he encouraged managers to meet and share experiences by asking questions regarding the new methods they heard about. This approach produced a radical improvement in productivity and spread to other organisations such as hospitals. Like many visionaries this brought conflict from the establishment as conventional lecture techniques were favoured by the educational institutions. Action learning is now commonplace in industry throughout the world. Instead of traditional teaching methods which focus on the presentation of information a group will pose questions to their colleagues that allow solutions to be developed in a process that incorporates reflection and problem solving. We have found this helpful in local problem-solving meetings when development is reviewed and the issues that seem insoluble are addressed. Some authorities have recommended the use of facilitators or coaches to guide group development but that is not mandatory.

Forming a Steering Group

The adoption of enhanced recovery should ideally be consultant led [2], with surgeons and anaesthetists taking the initiative. These clinical leaders must be able to present the evidence for change in a positive and inspirational manner. Another key to success is the formation of a steering group to ensure that a comprehensive pathway is developed and aligned to local needs. This group should include:

- Surgeon
- Anaesthetist
- Service manager

- Senior ward staff
- Pre-assessment staff
- Specialist nurse consultant (such as colorectal specialist nurse)
- Pain team representative
- Physiotherapist
- Nutritionist
- Occupational therapist
- Social care team representative
- Primary care representative
- Patient representative
- ER facilitator

It is essential that this group takes into consideration the needs of all stakeholders (including commissioners and other organisations or teams that collaborate or compete with the group). Groups that have experience of implementing ER in a relatively short timescale emphasise the importance of close cooperation between all the relevant departments and professions [3].

The role of the ER facilitator is to take the outcomes of the steering group and ensure that they are put into practice. Depending on the local circumstances, the facilitator could be a new, fixed term appointment specifically to introduce ER, or a secondment/re-grading for existing staff on a full or part-time basis (see Chap. 9 for more details).

The main aims of the steering group are:

- To evaluate the existing care pathway with respect to the established ER elements
- Agree on the aspects of the care pathway that need to change
- Create a business case to support any required investment or re-allocation of resources for change
- Identify the potential barriers to change
- Form an action plan to transform the care pathway
- Agree on outcome measures to record that will provide clear information on progress (or lack of it)
- Suggest methods to increase awareness of the new care pathway within the organisation/wider team
- Act as role models and inspire colleagues to adopt change

A series of operational groups should be formed to implement the changes suggested by the steering group. These groups will be linked to each aspect of the care pathway re-design. For example, if the steering group has identified a need to alter the information provided to patients before admission, a pre-assessment sub-group should be formed to ensure that this is implemented effectively. The ER facilitator should act as the link between each sub-group and report progress back to the steering group. Other sub-groups might be concerned with pain control, the provision of appropriate documentation and creation of an optimal environment for ER care. Most expert centres that have developed ER care have changed the ward environment by creating a dining area and, where possible, a lounge too. This encourages patients to be a more active participants in their recovery, walking to their meals rather than passively receiving them, trapped in their bed.

It is vital to have wider involvement with groups that may influence the care pathway. Optimising the patient's condition prior to admission for surgery is key and good relationships and information sharing with primary care and social care services is essential to ensure the success of ER. In addition to representation of these stakeholders on the steering group, awareness and education events must be scheduled before the programme is piloted. Formal seminars, informal social events and use of conventional and new media (such as local newspapers, DVDs, websites and blogs) can all be used to promote the new initiative.

The attitudes of team members have important implications for the success of the programme so it is essential that any reservations or reluctance are overcome before patients are recruited [2].

Writing a Business Case

Short-term investment may be needed to change the pathway (e.g. to employ an ER facilitator or project manager), to cover training for new skills (e.g. exercise testing), to purchase additional equipment (such as oesophageal Doppler and probes) and to fund awareness events and other educational opportunities.

Areas relating to referral that may require increased investment (dependant upon the existing situation locally) are optimising the health of the patient prior to admission and management of existing co-morbidities (such as diabetes, anaemia). Additional investment may also be related to pre-admission to support the promotion of informed decision-making, preoperative health and risk assessment and pre-operative therapy instruction (e.g. stoma care, physiotherapy). The immediate preoperative period may require additional support to allow carbohydrate loading and increased investment for intra-operative factors should cover minimal access surgery, use of regional or local anaesthetic, epidural anaesthetic or spinal blocks and individualised goal-directed fluid therapy. In the postoperative period, additional support may be needed for rapid hydration and nourishment, pain team management and other intensive therapy support (e.g. stoma care, physiotherapy). Finally, further resources could be allocated to the postdischarge period to cover telephone follow-up if that is deemed desirable.

These changes should see the following quality improvements:

- Better medical outcomes
- Reduced complications and decreased demand on ITU/HDU
- Improvements in patient satisfaction (through optimal management of expectations)
- Multi-disciplinary team working

In addition to the following productivity improvements:

- Appropriate length of stay results in improved efficiency
- Capacity will be released and activity may be increased

Note that ER may not necessarily result in cost savings, depending on the existing situation prior to implementing change [4]. Apart from the necessity to identify an ER facilitator, which may require investment if a reallocation of someone is not possible, most changes necessary to develop ER can be resource neutral if one looks critically at what is required, and takes advice from other centres. As the majority of patients leaving hospital in this programme also appear better than they used to be at discharge after conventional care, the concept that there will be increased health care requirements in the community is likely to be false. The concept that ER care reduces postoperative complications has been supported to date by the literature [5] but the number of patients studied is no more than 1,000. Further results will be keenly awaited to confirm that ER outside pioneering centres reduces complications and does not impact negatively on primary care.

Creation of a Care Pathway and Associated Literature

One of the key functions of the steering group is to create a new care pathway. This document should cover all aspects of patient care from admission to discharge, and be completed by the whole multi-professional team, with sections for patient comments or notes. Whilst it is possible to create a new pathway from scratch, many teams have found it helpful to adapt an existing pathway from another centre. As the pathway develops, or is amended, the ER facilitator relates the progress to each subgroup so that they can consider the impact on their own protocols and documentation. Examples of existing care pathways can be found at: http://www.dh.gov.uk/en/Healthcare/Electivecare/Enhancedrecovery/DH_115706

When considering the logistics of implementing the new pathway some thought must be given to covering absences of key staff and continuation of the pathway over weekends. Indeed, the first group to implement ER found that there was a marked, negative effect on the programme when the members of the research team were absent [6].

Setting Up an Audit of Outcomes and Monitoring the New Pathway

It is essential, when making changes to patient care pathways, that appropriate monitoring systems are in place to measure the effectiveness of these changes. Provided the correct aspects are measured, data entered correctly and monitored regularly, it will be possible for the steering group to gauge the success of the new protocol. In addition, any aspects that are not performing correctly can be picked up and corrective action taken. The Enhanced Recovery After Surgery (ERAS) Study

Group has undertaken a prospective audit in 1,035 patients, over a 3.5-year period and found that morbidity and mortality rates were lower for this cohort than previously published data for the same centres (prior to introduction of ER). Recording of compliance with the ER elements throughout the pathway enabled them to detect deviation from the protocol and to consider reasons for this variation [7].

As part of the ER Partnership Programme, a database has been developed for monitoring new ER sites/teams [8]. This consists of compulsory and optional fields covering demographics, admission details, patient experience, readmission, compliance with specific ER elements, complications, risk adjusters, postoperative morbidity score (POMS) and physiological and operative severity score for enumeration of mortality and morbidity (POSSUM).

The steering group should identify one individual with responsibility for data entry (usually the ER facilitator), who will report back to the group and take responsibility for instituting any suggested adjustments to the pathway.

Education

Several authors have stated the importance of increasing awareness and enthusiasm in all staff groups who will be working with the ER protocol [2, 9]. Education of colleagues is therefore a vital aspect for implementation of the programme. Many basic resources explaining the key elements of ER are now available on-line and some experienced sites provide courses or seminars. Comparison of the content between the various courses has yielded a series of key learning objectives [10]:

• Provide an overview to key principles of ER
• Emphasise pre-admission patient education and patient experience
• Outline the importance of preoperative optimisation of the patient
• Describe the anaesthetic aspects of ER
• Explain options for postoperative pain management
• Recount the impact of ER on ward nursing
• Describe roles of colorectal specialist nurse, stoma care practitioner, dietician and physiotherapist in relation to ER
• Together with their ER team, create short-term action plan for ER adoption

In addition to covering the above content, seminars at experienced centres provide a forum for discussion and informal advice, which is often invaluable to the novice group.

It is strongly recommended that a centre wishing to commence ER care take a multidisciplinary group to one of the training courses run on this subject. It is essential that education is delivered by a multidisciplinary faculty as different subspecialists are much more receptive to lectures from within their own specialty than those from others (Fig. 8.2). An example of this is the difficulty that certain clinicians have come across when they intrude on areas that are traditionally considered to be the preserve of other specialists, e.g., the exhortations by surgeons that an anaesthetist might consider changing the way they treat postoperative pain, or alter the type or

F. Carter and R.H. Kennedy

Fig. 8.2 Reflections on
multidisciplinary working

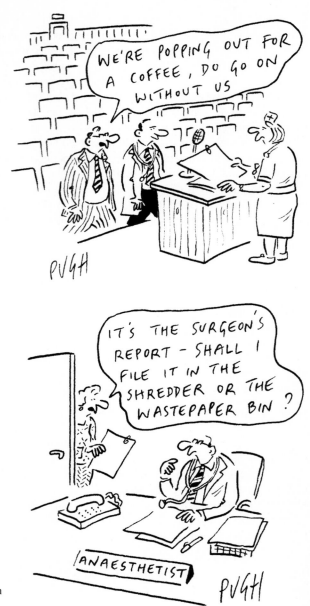

Fig. 8.3 Courtesy of Jonathan
Pugh

volume of fluid given to patients! Such interactions can be acrimonious 'turf' wars
that are counter-productive (Fig. 8.3), but with enlightened change management the
transition can be both hastened and made less confrontational. The other advantage
of a well-run multidisciplinary course is that all levels of staff being trained have the
opportunity to see the 'experts' being questioned in front of their peers and normally
by the end of the course contentious areas will have been thoroughly explored.

There will need to be a comprehensive programme of in-house education for local staff, which is tailored to the specific pathway and protocols that have been developed by the steering group. This education programme must take into account staff turnover and the need to re-educate at regular intervals [11]. The ER facilitator should take responsibility for delivery of this in-house teaching programme and must therefore have the necessary skills and abilities for this aspect of their role.

The importance of patient and relative (or carer) education cannot be over-emphasised. Indeed there is much evidence that setting realistic expectations and giving the patient ownership of their recovery has a positive impact on health outcomes [2]. There is a wealth of resources available on-line together with a range of video and DVD materials [12] that can explain the typical patient journey within an ERP. Inclusion of the relatives and carers will also ensure that the patient is well prepared and positive for their surgery and subsequent recovery. Planning for discharge in the pre-admission clinic and early exploration of medical or social factors that may hinder recovery should ensure better adherence to the pathway.

Embedding the New Care Pathway

It is essential that the steering group set out a clear set of expectations as the pathway is adopted and consider how best to select patients. Another key factor for success is having clearly defined discharge criteria, such as the ability to tolerate solid food, return to preoperative mobility and good pain management with oral analgesia [13]. Any refinements to the protocols resulting from initial experience should be put in place and further awareness and education events organised. Audit and monitoring of the outcomes must continue, with ongoing meetings of the steering group to assess progress and ensure safety and quality elements are being met. Any bottlenecks in the system (such as issues around early mobilisation and oral nutrition or introduction of epidural anaesthesia) must be tackled. The ongoing need to encourage the whole multidisciplinary team to adopt this change should not be underestimated [9].

Overcoming Barriers and Troubleshooting

A follow-up survey of 23 novice ER groups, who had previously attended an introductory seminar at Yeovil District Hospital, found that only 35% had subsequently implemented an ER pathway [10]. Further exploration of the reasons for the lack of progress highlighted a series of barriers to change that mirror the published evidence on the subject. These barriers can be broken down into three types: social, professional and organisational [14].

Examples of social barriers are where staff are uncomfortable when the new protocol requires them to change their normal routine and important local opinion leaders have a negative influence on behaviour (either due to disagreement with evidence base or obsolete knowledge). Other issues may arise when patients, or their relatives, expect a conventional type of care and this can often be tackled via positive reports in local press and other media. In addition, current training programmes, such as higher surgical training or nurse training courses may not include ER as best practice and the new protocols may not be advocated by national organisations, industry, etc. Half of the novice groups followed up after the Yeovil course said that absence of a key member of staff or opinion leader was the main reason that the programme had stalled. Other articles have stressed the importance of the whole multidisciplinary team working together to improve patient management [2, 9].

Barriers relating to the professional context could be when staff may feel that results from literature could not be replicated in their own workplace or the overload of clinical evidence may cause difficulties with decision making. Specific staff groups tend to raise professional issues and present barriers to the adoption of ER:

• Consultant anaesthetists and surgeons
• Senior management
• Nursing staff

The anaesthetist has control over many vital aspects of the ER pathway and must move from an 'anonymous technician in the operating theatre', to becoming a 'visible perioperative medical specialist' outside theatre [2]. It is essential that the key anaesthetic elements are agreed upon and an appropriate anaesthetic care pathway is developed, with implementation monitored.

Many centres report initial difficulties with convincing their surgical colleagues to adopt ER with the typical reasons for reluctance being [2, 15]:

• Pressure of existing workload, need to meet cancer targets
• ER will increase risk of complications and readmissions
• Some patients do not want to have a short hospital stay
• Wards do not have the resources to support ER
• Risk of increased burden on primary care when patients discharged too soon
• Individuals are unconvinced by the available evidence base.

Thus it is important that a clinical champion and senior management provide support and evidence to refute each of these incorrect assumptions, so that ER is accepted as the optimal standard of care in colorectal surgery.

Restrictions in finances and logistical support can cripple the implementation of a new programme. Senior hospital managers must be convinced of the need for change and the likely benefits so that they can support the clinical champion, ER steering group and co-ordinator to implement the new programme.

It is often difficult to convince nursing staff of the benefits of change when the new care pathway appears to go against the existing culture of care. In addition, time pressures and lack of staff are often mentioned as inhibitors to adoption of a new programme. Any inconsistencies in opinion or practice from senior medical staff will create confusion and uncertainty for nursing staff on the ward. This lack of confidence in the care pathway will ultimately be transferred to the patient. Involving key nursing staff in the steering group and having strong leadership from the clinical champion and ER facilitator can counteract most of the issues raised above. Provision of adequate resources by senior management will also overcome inadequate staff numbers or other resources.

Organisational barriers to change include financial constraints (e.g. silo funding for specific aspects related to ER), pressure of work, staff shortages, inefficient audit of performance or lack of other resources. There may also be a perception of potential liability such as risks of increased complaints due to high readmission rates or an increased burden on primary care. Finally, there are the perceived expectations of patients; perhaps they are expecting traditional care pathways and we are unsure of the impact of ER on relatives or carers. Of the centres followed up after the Yeovil courses, 72% indicated that lack of resources, financial or administrative support impeded their adoption of ER [10].

Many centres have attempted to adopt ER by gradually incorporating certain elements or involving various disciplines. This can often lead to disillusionment when improvements in patient outcome are difficult to discern. A better approach is to formulate a comprehensive care pathway, involving a steering group, which represents all members of the multidisciplinary team, with a planned audit of results.

Finally, the importance of ensuring that the ward environment is conducive to an ER programme should not be underestimated. Important aspects of ER such as postoperative mobilisation and encouraging patient independence, with supported access to food and self-care facilities require a rehabilitation unit environment. Steps should be taken, where physically and financially possible, to create a patient-friendly environment which supports ER [16].

Summary

This chapter has highlighted the main elements required for success in adoption of ER care and discussed how to get started, step by step. Strong clinical leadership, good multiprofessional collaboration and involvement of all key stakeholders are all vital. Testing and subsequent embedding of the new pathway, together with promotion and educational events, have been described. Groups intending to set out on this journey should be aware of the potential barriers to change and take steps to tackle these issues at an early stage.

Acknowledgement With greatful thanks to MRJ. Pugh for figs. 8.2–8.3.

References

1. Kotter JP. Leading change. Boston: Harvard Business School Press; 1996. Product no 7471.
2. Kahokehr A, Sammour T, Zargar-Shoshtari K, Thompson L. Implementation of ERAS and how to overcome the barriers. Int J Surg. 2009;7:16–9.
3. Jottard KJC, Van Berlo C, Jeuken L, Dejong C. Changes in outcome during implementation of a fast-track colonic surgery project in a university-affiliated general teaching hospital: advantages reached with ERAS over a 1-year period. Dig Surg. 2008;25:335–8.

4. Driver A. Supporting the implementation of enhanced recovery. 2011. Available at: http://www.dh.gov.uk/en/Healthcare/Electivecare/Enhancedrecovery/DH_115793. Accessed 3 May 2011.
5. Varadhan KK, Neal KR, Dejong CH, Fearon KC, Ljungqvist O, Lobo DN. The enhanced recovery after surgery (ERAS) pathway for patients undergoing major elective open colorectal surgery: a meta-analysis of randomized controlled trials. Clin Nutr. 2010;29(4):434–40.
6. Basse L, Thorbol JE, Lossl K, Kehlet H. Colonic surgery with accelerated rehabilitation or conventional care. Dis Colon Rectum. 2004;47:271–8.
7. Hendry PO, Hausel J, Nygren J, Lassen K, Dejong CHC, Ljungqvist O, et al. Determinants of outcome after colorectal resection within an enhanced recovery programme. Br J Surg. 2009;96:197–205.
8. Enhanced Recovery Programme Toolkit. 2011. Available at: http://www.natcansatmicrosite.net/enhancedrecovery/. Accessed 3 May 2011.
9. Polle SW, Wind J, Fuhring J, Hofland J, Gouma DJ, Bemelman WA. Implementation of a fast-track perioperative care programme: what are the difficulties? Dig Surg. 2007;24:441–9.
10. Carter F. Achieving widespread adoption of colorectal enhanced recovery in England: learning from the current UK centres. Discussion document for Enhanced Recovery Partnership Programme, July 2009. Available at http://www.enhancedrecoveryhub/2112.html. Accessed 4 May 2011.
11. Maessen J, Dejong CH, Hausel J, Nygren J, Lassen K, Andersen J, et al. A protocol is not enough to implement an enhanced recovery programme. Br J Surg. 2007;94:224–31.
12. Francis N, Carter F. "Bowel Cancer: A Patient's Journey". 2009 NHS Training for Innovation Patient Education DVD: http://www.tfistore.co.uk/brands/Yeovil-District-Hospital-NHS-Foundation-Trust.html.
13. Wind J, Polle SW, Fung Kon Jin PHP, Dejong CHC, von Meyenfeldt MF, Ubbink DT, et al. Systematic review of enhanced recovery programmes in colonic surgery. Br J Surg. 2006;93:800–9.
14. Grol R, Grimshaw J. From best evidence to best practice: effective implementation of change in patients' care. Lancet. 2003;362:1225–30.
15. Walter CJ, Smith A, Guillou P. Perceptions of the application of fast-track surgical principles by general surgeons. Ann R Coll Surg Engl. 2006;88:191–5.
16. Pattison HM, Robertson CE. The effect of ward design on the well being of post-operative patients. J Adv Nurs. 1996;23:820–6.

Chapter 9
The Role of the Enhanced Recovery Facilitator

Jane P. Bradley Hendricks and Fiona Carter

Introduction

The key to ensuring successful implementation of enhanced recovery is engagement, commitment and involvement of the multidisciplinary team across the local health community. Enhanced recovery (ER) will fail without teamwork and the role of the ER facilitator is paramount to the success of the programme [1]. The ER facilitator must have access to all the key members of the team and be able to convince reluctant colleagues of the importance of change. Since this ER programme crosses all areas of the patient journey, the facilitator will need to have a good understanding of the issues related to each aspect of care. The role of the facilitator is not to give the care at each patient episode but to oversee the programme and ensure that it is carried out in each department.

Developing the Role

This is the responsibility of the ER steering board, which will be aware of the current skills mix within the existing team and of individuals who would be suitable to take on this additional role. The board will need to consider whether this should be a new appointment, a secondment or a full or part-time change of role or responsibility. If the person is well known in the organisation this can also be a useful attribute,

J.P.B. Hendricks (✉)
Department of General Surgery, Colchester General Hospital, Colchester, Essex, UK
e-mail: jane.hendricks@colchesterhospital.nhs.uk

F. Carter
Yeovil Academy, Yeovil District Hospital NHS Foundation Trust, Yeovil, Somerset, UK

N. Francis et al. (eds.), *Manual of Fast Track Recovery for Colorectal Surgery,*
Enhanced Recovery, DOI 10.1007/978-0-85729-953-6_9,
© Springer-Verlag London Limited 2012

although not essential. The facilitator needs to work across the multidisciplinary team and be involved in all areas of patient care [1]. Appendix 9.1 provides a sample job description.

Line management for an ER facilitator should involve a person that can reflect the multidisciplinary nature of the role, for example the service manager for surgery. Should this person be someone without a nursing background, there is also a requirement for line management from a senior nurse for accountability for the nursing aspect of the work.

Once the appointment process is complete, the new ER facilitator may need to undertake some professional development to help them in their new role. Attendance at study days or seminars, run at various expert sites across the UK, is often very helpful and many ER teams prefer to attend such courses together, ensuring a level-playing field of knowledge [1, 2]. It is essential that each team member has a good understanding of the involvement of their colleagues within the team and the ER facilitator can help to promote this. Experienced teams may welcome observers for a short period of time, so that a new ER facilitator can see an ER pathway in action. There are also a range of resources available to assist with pathway development, patient information and data collection [3].

Identifying individuals to work with from each speciality, outpatients, physiotherapy, dietetics, pharmacy, the ward, theatres, pain team, etc. is essential. Each individual must be prepared to adopt the necessary changes to their protocols [4, 5]. The hospital management must be supportive as the co-operation of the bed managers for example is essential (both to adopt the concept of admission on the day of surgery and postoperative placement of the patients onto a specific surgical ward).

The ER facilitator needs to have a full understanding of the programme and be able to answer a variety of questions with confidence. This is essential if they are to gain the support of their colleagues.

Getting Started

In units where there are more than one colorectal surgeon, it is extremely helpful if all the consultants agree to have their patients managed in the same way; this applies pre-, peri- and postoperatively. Enlisting the co-operation of all the consultants to sign up to the same protocols will ensure that the programme will be more successful, as all the other members of the team are working towards the same end [4]. This is also true for the consultant anaesthetists who are responsible for the patients, and having a written protocol also helps in training junior colleagues. The role of the ER facilitator is extremely important to ensure all this is put in place. In theory with evidence-based medicine, enforcing this practice should not be difficult. However in practice, streamlining everyone's practice is probably the hardest aspect to achieve. The rolling out of the programme will not succeed if this is not considered seriously.

In the early stages, regular ER team meetings are essential to ensure that any issues are resolved and potential problems can be dealt with. Initially this could be on a monthly basis, changing the day of the week to ensure everyone can attend.

The ER facilitator will be responsible for creation of the patient documentation taking advice from all members of the multidisciplinary team. This will include the pathway and any documentation that the patient requires as part of their care. There should be an agreed time frame for this to be updated and reviewed. It should all be passed through the patient public information governance committee before it is circulated amongst patients. Once this has been agreed, it is useful to pilot the paperwork and gain some feedback before agreeing on the final documentation.

Utilising patient information, guidelines and pathways from other trusts is actively encouraged to try to alleviate the 'reinventing the wheel' scenario [3]. Most National Health Scheme (NHS) trusts are happy to share their documentation, but individuals should always get their explicit permission to avoid any conflict in the future or accusations of plagiarism.

Managing patient expectations of their hospital stay is often quoted as an essential factor in the success of an ER programme. One key aspect to get this right is written and verbal patient information about the ER pathway. Giving patients' ownership of their recovery is very empowering and this positive mental attitude will have a beneficial effect on their postoperative rehabilitation [6].

Patients should only be discharged once they meet clearly defined criteria:

- Managing well with oral painkillers
- Tolerating a normal diet
- Able to mobilise well and undertake normal activities
- Managing their stoma independently (if applicable)

The discharge information must include 24/7 phone details for a senior member of the ER team, together with clear details on when to contact the team for support. The important factor here is to discuss with the patient how they should feel and give them sufficient written information to back this up. One of the simplest ways of doing this is to tell the patient that each day they should get better and better; if they feel worse then they should contact the surgical team. Realistically most patients that go home on day 4 or 5 are well, those who are going to develop an anastomotic leak are usually not well from day 2 and in general they are not "quite right" and therefore will not meet the discharge criteria in a shorter time frame.

Each ER team will investigate the best way of ensuring 24/7 contact; this could be via a mobile phone that is primarily carried by a senior member of the ER team, preferably the facilitator. In this case the facilitator should have an overview and be familiar with the patient.

There are a variety of ways that the ER phone can be managed, for example it can be held by the ER facilitator during the day and passed to the on-call surgical registrar out of hours. Other establishments may have the facilitator hold the phone from Monday to Friday and then pass to the on call team at the weekend. If this is the case they have to ensure that, if they are not being paid to hold the phone out of hours, they are covered to give information to patients in time that they are not actually at work. This can be addressed by adding it to their job description and therefore they are covered by vicarious liability. The person holding the phone must know what questions to ask and what to do with the information received. Trying to discern whether a patient has a urinary tract infection or an anastomotic leak is important, as you do not want the patient to be re-admitted unless it is absolutely necessary. On the other hand, you do not want to miss the signs of an anastomotic leak and reassure the patient that they are fine when in fact they are not.

Establishing an area or ward space where the patient can be assessed by a senior person in a short space of time can be problematic and it is worth doing the homework in advance [7]. The number of times that this facility will be used will be minimal, in which case it may be acceptable to use the emergency and assessment ward triage area. Another alternative is to identify a treatment room on the ward that they have been discharged from. Cultivating a good working relationship with bed managers may also help as they will quickly be able to identify a bed space that you can use for a short period of time, whilst you are assessing the patient. It cannot be emphasised at this point that if you have a robust discharge plan in place, the times that you will need to use this facility will be minimal. However, if the patients are unwell they need to be reviewed promptly by a senior member of the emergency team; this should be agreed by all the surgical consultants and passed onto the registrars.

Another aspect of the role is to ensure that liaison is carried out with primary care. This is important both prior to the admission for surgery and post-discharge. It is essential to allay any fears that primary care may have regarding early discharge and managing complications. It is important to stress that the ER team would much prefer direct contact with the patient should problems arise between discharge and follow-up. Once you have all the systems in place, before you roll out the programme, it is useful to invite local GPs, practice nurses and district nurses to an information event, taking this opportunity to share with them your aspirations and what you are hoping to achieve and more importantly what you would like them to assist you with.

Once you have run the programme for 6 months or so, it is useful to invite them for another event to share the results with them. This helps to bridge the gap between primary and secondary care and also gives each side the opportunity to share any concerns they may have.

Managing Care

Outpatient Clinic

Patients are given a substantial amount of information at the outpatient clinic; usually all they will remember is the diagnosis and that they need an operation. Often the next question is how long will I spend in hospital; this is the appropriate time to introduce the concept of the ER. Very little of the information will be retained, so backing it up with written information is important. They can then read this later on and have a better opportunity to digest the information. The programme will be reinforced at each stage of their journey. Meeting the ER facilitator may be appropriate at this stage or the specialist nurse dealing with them may be able to deliver the information. The consultant should also mention the concept of ER whilst discussing all aspects of their forthcoming surgery.

Preadmission Clinic

Setting up a preadmission service, or streamlining one that is already in place can be one of the first serious tasks to initiate. Admission on the day of surgery will only be successful if a thorough and comprehensive preadmission is carried out and must involve all members of the MDT [3].

Timing of preadmission can be difficult. The current fashion is for everyone to go straight to preadmission once it has been determined that they need surgery. In reality this is neither practical nor feasible. Certainly for major surgery, patients may have just been told that they have cancer and need an operation. This is all the information they can take onboard and need to go away and share it with other members of their family or friends. They need time to start to formulate all the questions that they wish to have answered.

Inviting them back for a preadmission at a pre-determined time is often better for everyone, but primarily this has the patient's best interests at heart; they will also have the opportunity to invite a partner, relative or carer to come with them.

Clearly it is not possible for the ER facilitator to deliver every aspect of the programme, therefore the preadmission staff should be fully informed about the programme and be able to deliver this information to the patient [1–5]. They should have access to the facilitator if the patients have questions that they cannot answer. The information that they are given verbally at this time should be backed up by written information. The patient should also have the contact details of the ER facilitator should they have questions once they have left the hospital.

It is also useful to try and time preadmission clinics when the consultant anaesthetist is available to see the patient. This in practice can be problematic, but there are a number of ways around the problem. If the preadmission area is geographically close to the theatre suite, then the anaesthetist may be able to come and see the patient. Often there is a floating anaesthetist who will cover whilst they go and see the patient. If this is not possible, the patient can be asked to wait for a little while until the anaesthetist is available and this time can be used to cover all the other aspects of preadmission as well as having bloods taken, spriometry, ECG etc. If they are unable to wait, or need a more in-depth consultation, then it may be appropriate to book them a separate anaesthetic appointment. Those patients who are obviously unfit should be referred and seen by the anaesthetist prior to coming to preadmission.

Day of Surgery Admission

In the ideal situation for day of surgery admission is a purpose built area that is staffed Monday to Friday from 7 a.m. to 4 p.m., and is closed at weekends. This is beneficial to the hospital as it saves money on staffing out of hours, and is beneficial to the staff as they only work during the week and on an early shift.

The patient should come into the hospital at 7 a.m. and the final documentation completed before they leave the ward for theatre at 8 a.m. The number of beds provided by the admission area will depend on the number of theatres requiring the service. It is only important to have the first patient for each list in a bed and there must be a good system in place to replenish the beds as they go to theatre.

A room should also be available where the anaesthetists and the surgeon can see and consent the subsequent patients on the list, if this has not been done already.

Another option is that you can have trolleys in the admission ward and the patients that are able walk to theatre with an escort and are placed in a bed once they get to theatre or a holding bay if there is one available.

The bed managers must have a working knowledge of the number of elective admissions expected. This will enable them to plan ahead and allocate beds in the appropriate ward.

Other hospitals have a 5-day stay ward where the beds are ring-fenced for elective surgery. In this instance, someone needs to be responsible for mapping the patients through the available beds on a weekly basis. This is often multi-speciality and can be complex to arrange, however with coordination from all the various specialities it is a feasible and workable option. Those patients who will obviously require a longer than a 5-day stay (or need to stay over the weekend) will need to be accommodated on the appropriate long stay ward.

Surgery

The ER facilitator must have a good working knowledge of what happens to the patient in the theatre. The theatre team are primarily involved with the surgery but should have a working knowledge of what an ER programme entails. It is not essential that they come to all meetings as the time the patient spends in theatre will not change dramatically as long as laparoscopic or minimal access surgery is already used. If this is not the case, and if the organisation is introducing laparoscopy, this is indeed a very substantial piece of work to undertake. It may be appropriate to undertake the change in surgical intervention first and think about the implementation of an ER programme at a later stage.

Recovery

It is often perceived that many patients will require ITU or HDU facilities after surgery, however in reality this is rarely the case [1, 5]. A better option for the patient is transfer to the recovery room and for them to spend an extended time there before transfer back to the ward. This can be anything from 2 to 4 h to ensure that the patient is stable and pain free before return to the ward. All patients should be offered something to drink to encourage oral fluid intake and then the intravenous fluids may be discontinued if appropriate.

Postoperative Recovery

The patients should go back to a specific ward area that has a complete understanding of all the postoperative aspects of ER. Having flow charts and protocols (see Appendix 9. 2 for examples) that are agreed by all members of the MDT is essential at this point. These should be part of the patient care pathway or can be laminated and placed at the end of the patient's bed. The immediate postoperative period is fraught with problems trying to ensure that patients do not get given too much intravenous fluid. Treating low blood pressure in patients with epidurals for example is a complex issue, and in some extreme circumstances the patient may have to be transferred to HDU for the administration of vasoconstrictors to correct the physiological response of the epidural [5, 8].

The patient should be seen by the surgical team at least twice a day and this will include the ER facilitator. The morning ward round determines the plan of care for the day (this should be reinforcing the protocol) and the afternoon ward round should ensure that all the morning plans have been successfully completed, review the blood tests and determine the fluid regime for the next 12 h. It can be helpful if the patients are cared for by separate teams and the ward round becomes a generic elective colorectal ward round where all patients are seen by the same team. This helps to streamline the care and ensure that each patient receives the same standard of care based upon the same principles [1, 4, 5].

The date for discharge will have been planned with the patient in preadmission and, providing the surgery went as planned and there have been no postoperative complications, this is the date that everyone works to.

On discharge the patient will be given written information that will address some of their questions and most importantly they will be given the mobile number of the facilitator, so they have a way back into the system should this be required.

Data Collection

The ER facilitator will be responsible for data collection of outcomes and compliance to ER elements. This is essential as it will inform you as to the success or failure of the programme [1, 5, 9]. It is also important to involve the patients in this process also.

Patient involvement can be in the form of telephone follow-ups on the day after discharge or by completion of patient satisfaction questionnaires or patient diaries.

This should encompass their view of the service and how it was delivered, what they felt good about, what they disliked, what they felt could be improved, etc. This is essential and is part of the quality of the patient experience, which should be at the centre of all aspects of patient care.

Evaluation of the ER Programme

The collection of data will also allow you to evaluate the programme and identify areas that can be improved. This is very valuable feedback to the clinical team and is also a good benchmarking exercise, assisting with the provision of services and planning work for the next financial year.

Appendix 9.1: Sample Job Description for Enhanced Recovery Facilitator

Title

Enhanced Recovery Nurse

Grade

Band 7

Key Relationships

Line Manager, Matron, Ward Sisters and Ward staff, Consultants & Teams, Anaesthetists, Physiotherapists, Occupational Therapist, Acute Pain Team, POA, Admissions, Surgical Site Infection Nurse, Enhanced Recovery Nurses from other specialities, Consultant Secretaries, Outpatients, Theatres staff, Business Manager, Social Worker, Pharmacist, Patient's & Relatives.

Job Summary

The post holder will be responsible for:

- Developing the role of the Enhanced Recovery Nurse, caring for patients undergoing elective surgical procedures.

- To manage the care of the patients in the Enhanced Recovery Programme.
- To develop training programmes for Ward Staff and other disciplines in the Enhanced Recovery Programme.

Main Duties and Responsibilities

Clinical Practice and Practice Development

1. The post holder will create and sustain key relationships with the Multi Disciplinary Team, (MDT) the Primary Healthcare professionals and social care to support the interface between primary and secondary services and provide expertise regarding the management of surgical procedures and the needs of patient's pre and post operatively.
2. Identify patients that may have the correct criteria for the Enhanced Recovery Programme and promote appropriate timely referral to the MDT, Primary Healthcare Professionals and liaise with other health and social care providers to promote high standards in discharge planning and remapping patient pathways.
3. To work consistently and autonomously as a clinical expert in the post of Enhanced Recovery Nurse.
4. To undertake assessment of patients cared for in the Enhanced Recovery Programme, to ensure their suitability and that all potential risks are identified and managed.
5. Provide accurate written and verbal information for patients and relatives pre operatively and promote health education.
6. Liaise with other health care professionals, documenting the ongoing care requirements and communicating any changes.
7. Ensure good communication both written and verbal between all members of the multi disciplinary team, patients and relatives.
8. Be a point of contact/professional liaison for all the members of the multi disciplinary team.
9. Be a patient advocate.
10. Ensure accurate and comprehensive patient records are kept and that all members of the multidisciplinary team are using the correct documentation.
11. Ensure patients receive all the relevant information, appointment and discharge documentation on discharge. Provide a telephone follow up service once discharged, be able to provide effective telephone post-operative advice.
12. Demonstrate appropriate behaviour in stressful and difficult situations. Support junior members of staff encountering difficult situations.
13. Maintain and encourage high standards of practice, challenging those who do not. Ensure corrective action is taken.
14. Promote evidence-based decision-making.
15. Demonstrate counseling skills for patients and relatives, being supportive when they receive bad news.

Service Development and Management

1. Actively support the implementation of the Enhanced Recovery Programme to improve patient care.
2. Assist in the development of protocols and pathways, which are evidence based to manage the assessment and treatment of patients on the Enhanced Recovery Programme.
3. Provide expert advice to Senior Nurses, Consultants and the MDT to secure quality improvements within the organization and across boundaries.
4. Prepare and write regular reports on the outcomes of the Enhanced Recovery Programme for presentation to the Division.
5. Maintain a database for all patients on the Enhanced Recovery Programme.
6. Participate in presentations in the Trust and for outside organisations in the Enhanced Recovery Programme.
7. Keep up to date with developments in the service, introducing new ideas to improve patient care.
8. Develop some understanding of the commissioning process to support and inform service redesign across the local health economy.
9. Attend relevant meetings providing information as requested.

Research and Audit

1. Ensure care being provided is evidence based
2. Develop relevant audits to support the development of the Enhanced Recovery Programme and implement recommendations to ensure sustainability of the service.
3. Monitor standard of care being delivered. Research and lead on improvements of care.
4. Audit outcomes of the Enhanced Recovery Programme, benchmarking other Trusts undertaking the Enhanced Recovery Programme.
5. Implement and maintain Surgical Site Infection Surveillance as determined by the Health Protection Agency, liaising with the Trust Surgical Site Infection Nurse.

Professional/Education and Training Role

1. To promote the role of the Enhanced Recovery Nurse in the Trust.
2. To act as a role model and provide leadership to junior staff.
3. Provide guidance and act as a resource for members of staff, supporting and motivating them.

4. Provide day-to-day guidance for nursing and junior medical staff.
5. Formulate a training programme for nursing and junior medical staff. Promote an active learning environment.
6. Actively participate in appraisals, identifying training requirements and maintaining competencies.
7. Adhere to the NMC Code of Conduct and Trust Policies.

Financial Responsibility

1. Be aware of financial constraints and savings programmes.
2. Promote cost saving initiatives.
3. Consider financial implications when prescribing and implementing treatments.

Risk Management

1. In conjunction with the MDT, set and review standards, protocols and procedures, ensuring remedial action taken if standards fall below acceptable level.
2. Adhere to Trust policy by facilitating and using clinical risk evaluation and incident reporting.
3. Take responsibility to resolve or remove risk where possible, notifying and working with Manager when not possible.

Note

The duties and responsibilities outlined in this job description although comprehensive are not definitive and you may be required to perform other duties at the request of your manager.

This job description is designed to reflect duties currently incorporated in this post. These may change in the light of changes in the service provided by the Trust. Any such changes will be fully discussed with the post holder.

Person Specification Form

Job title: Enhanced Recovery
Grade: Band 7

Factors	Essential requirements	Desirable requirements
Qualifications	• First level RGN	• Independent nurse prescriber
	• Mentorship & Preceptorship or ENB 998	• Degree in nursing or working towards
	• Good written and spoken English	
	• IT skills	
	• Evidence of continued Professional development	
Knowledge	• Extensive current working and theoretical knowledge of surgical nursing	
Experience	• Three years senior nurse experience in surgical nursing	• Experience of presenting to groups of staff
	• Experience of managing a team of nurses	• Experience of counselling
	• Experience of research and implementation of new practices	• Experience of Nurse Led Clinics
	• Experience of developing and writing integrated care pathways	• Nurse led discharges
		• Working in the community
Skills and ability	• Effective communication skills	• Previous experience of undertaking audits
	• Good leadership qualities	• Evidence of leading change management
	• Experience of teaching	• Implementation of new ways of working
	• Experience in change management	
	• Able to work autonomously and as part of a team	
	• Ability to write reports	
	• Ability to work across boundaries	
	• Ability to cope with stress and work under pressure	
	• Works under own initiative	
	• Car driver	
Personal qualities	• Motivated	
	• Approachable	
	• Good interpersonal skills	
	• Organised	
	• Calm & objective	
	• Open to change with the ability to adapt to rapidly changing environments	
	• Able to update and manage own development	

Appendix 9.2: Sample Flow Charts and Protocols

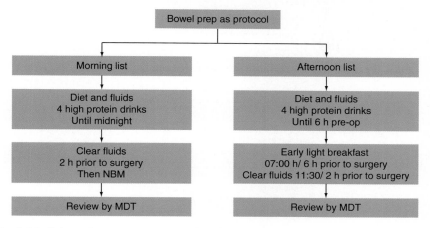

Fig. A.9.1 Enhanced recovery programme day of admission

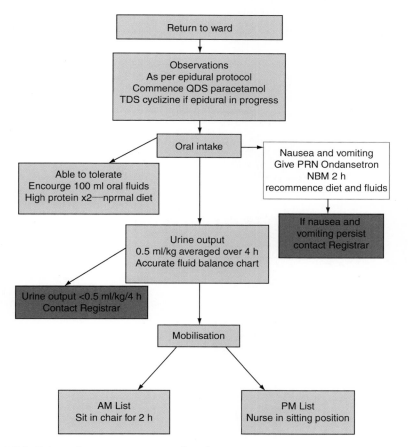

Fig. A.9.2 Enhanced recovery programme day of surgery

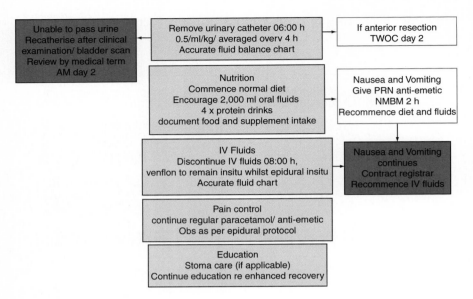

Fig. A.9.3 Postoperative day 1

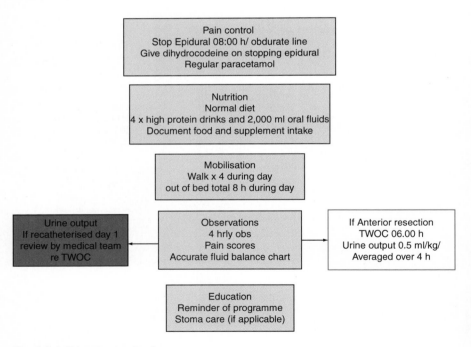

Fig. A.9.4 Postoperative day 2

Fig. A.9.5 Postoperative day 3

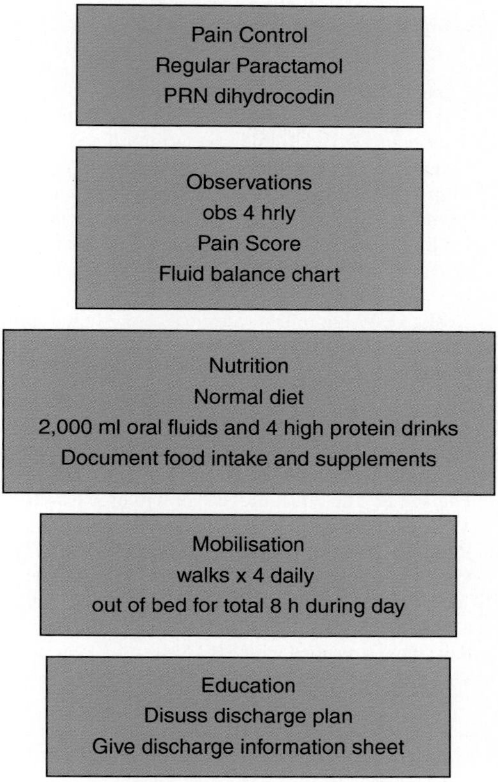

Pain Control
Regular Paractamol
PRN dihydrocodin

Observations
obs 4 hrly
Pain Score
Fluid balance chart

Nutrition
Normal diet
2,000 ml oral fluids and 4 high protein drinks
Document food intake and supplements

Mobilisation
walks x 4 daily
out of bed for total 8 h during day

Education
Disuss discharge plan
Give discharge information sheet

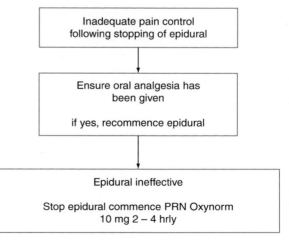

Inadequate pain control
following stopping of epidural

Ensure oral analgesia has
been given

if yes, recommence epidural

Epidural ineffective

Stop epidural commence PRN Oxynorm
10 mg 2 – 4 hrly

Fig. A.9.6 Postoperative pain
control

References

1. Evans J, Kennedy RH. Enhanced recovery after surgery, chapter 12. In: Kingsnorth AN, Bowley DM, editors. Fundamentals of surgical practice: a preparation guide for the MRCS intercollegiate exam. 3rd ed. Cambridge: Cambridge University Press; 2011.
2. Carter F. Achieving widespread adoption of colorectal enhanced recovery in England: learning from the current UK centres. Discussion document for enhanced recovery partnership programme, July 2009. http://www.enhancedrecoveryhub/2112.html. Accessed 4 May 2011.
3. On-line resources to support spread and adoption of enhanced recovery provided by the UK Department of Health. http://www.dh.gov.uk/en/Healthcare/Electivecare/Enhancedrecovery/ DH_115706
4. Kehlet H, Wilmore DW. Surgical care – how can new evidence be applied to clinical practice. Colorectal Dis. 2010;12(1):2–4.
5. Maessen J, Dejong CH, Hausel J, Nygren J, Lassen K, Andersen J, et al. A protocol is not enough to implement an enhanced recovery programme. Br J Surg. 2007;94:224–31.
6. Khoo CK, Vickery CJ, Forsyth N, Vinall NS, Eyre-Brook IA. A prospective randomized controlled trial of multimodal perioperative management protocol in patients undergoing elective colorectal resection for cancer. Ann Surg. 2007;245(6):867–72.
7. Pattison R. The effect of ward design on the well being of post-operative patients. J Adv Nurs. 1996;23:820–6.
8. Polle SW, Wind J, Fuhring J, Hofland J, Gouma DJ, Bemelman WA. Implementation of a fast-track perioperative care programme: what are the difficulties? Dig Surg. 2007;24:441–9.
9. Jottard KJC, Van Berlo C, Jeuken L, Dejong C. Changes in outcome during implementation of a fast-track colonic surgery project in a university-affiliated general teaching hospital. Advantages reached with ERAS over a 1-year period. Dig Surg. 2008;25:335–8.

Chapter 10
Success and Failure in Colorectal Enhanced Recovery

Nader Francis, Andrew Allison, and Jonathan Ockrim

Introduction

Enhanced recovery (ER) after surgery programmes should succeed in improving the quality of care and reducing the length of stay for the majority of patients undergoing colorectal surgery. A minority of patients however are perceived to fail by these measures and it is in these patients that we see some of the challenges and limitations faced by ER programmes.

The success or failure of an ER programme should be defined not on the terms of the clinician, nurse, bed manager or accountant (although these are all important), but ultimately on the patient's terms. The individual patient's understanding, expectations, anxieties and physical function all need to be addressed in an ER programme. The focus on 'success' in ER should therefore move away from the speed of discharge and be directed more towards the quality of care and the recovery from the patient's perspective.

Measuring Success and Failure in ER

For discussion purposes, the success and failure of ER are examined in this chapter under the following measures:

- Outcome measures such as length of stay, readmission and complications
- Functional recovery and patient satisfaction
- Compliance with or deviation from the ER protocol

N. Francis (✉) • A. Allison
Department of Surgery, Yeovil District Hospital, Yeovil, Somerset, UK

J. Ockrim
Department of Surgery, Yeovil District Hospital, NHS Foundation Trust, Yeovil, Somerset, UK

N. Francis et al. (eds.), *Manual of Fast Track Recovery for Colorectal Surgery*,
Enhanced Recovery, DOI 10.1007/978-0-85729-953-6_10,
© Springer-Verlag London Limited 2012

Outcome Measures in ER

Up to date, four systematic reviews on the outcome measures of ER following bowel resection have supported the use of ER over traditional post-operative care in terms of a shorter post-operative length of stay, lower complication rates and acceptable readmission rates [1–4].

The original ER programme as described by Kehlet resulted in a reduction of median post-operative length of stay following open colonic resection to 2 days [5]. Since then other institutions and collaborating groups have found practical difficulties in reproducing such excellent results with some quoting instead a median post-operative stay following open surgery of 5 days [6]. There can be several reasons to account for these differences. The original Kehlet paper was a feasibility study examining a small group of 60 partly selected patients undergoing segmental colectomy with transverse incisions and epidural analgesia and who were deemed fit for planned discharge 2 days after surgery so that there was no delay in their functional recovery. In contrast, subsequent studies have examined non-selected patients undergoing more extensive open resections including anterior resection with transverse or midline incisions with or without epidural. The Enhanced Recovery After Surgery (ERAS) collaboration group [6] examined such a heterogeneous group of 425 patients (that included more extensive resections but who also had epidural analgesia) and demonstrated that discharge occurred at a median of 5 days postoperatively. Nevertheless, a median LOS of 5 days for all elective colorectal resection should be considered a success, considering the national median LOS across England was 9 days in 2009 according to the National Bowel Cancer Audit Programme (NBOCP 2009).

Comparable mortality rates but significant reductions in post-operative morbidities have been documented in systematic reviews comparing conventional post-operative care to the ER protocol [1–4]. Furthermore, these differences can be demonstrated upon the introduction of an ER protocol to a non-established unit [7]. It is currently not clear which combinations of the ER components (early enteral nutrition, early mobilisation, epidural, opiate-sparing analgesia or a restrictive intravenous fluid policy) derive maximum benefit for the individual patient with their own co-morbidities. Until such a time, the best chances of success in terms of low mortality and morbidity appear to come by applying the complete ER protocol.

Functional Recovery and Patient Satisfaction in ER

Functional recovery can be measured by either gastrointestinal (GI) function, patient mobility score or health-related quality of life assessment tools. GI function has been shown to return to normality significantly quicker using ER. This is variously attributed to early oral nutrition, the use of epidural and or opioid sparing analgesia and early mobilisation [8–10]. A restrictive fluids policy has a similar positive effect [11]. Although gastrointestinal function shows a quicker functional recovery following laparoscopic surgery [12, 13] and when laparoscopic surgery is combined with ER [14] the benefits to date are not clear when laparoscopic surgery is compared to ER [15, 16]. Similarly, it is difficult to demonstrate a clear benefit of laparoscopic ER over open ER in terms of patient's physical functional recovery (mobilisation) for the small study sizes conducted to date [16].

A systematic review [17] was carried out to address whether early discharge within ER had any deleterious effect on quality of life and patient satisfaction in comparison to conventional recovery. Given the limited available data to date (only ten small studies), ER does not adversely influence quality of life or psychomotor functions such as sleep quality, pain and fatigue levels after surgery. Moreover, there is some evidence that fatigue and pain may be less in the early post-operative period when ER pathways are used. Patients appear to be equally satisfied with ER and conventional recovery.

Compliance in ER

Within the framework set out by the ERAS collaboration group and more recently by the Enhanced Recovery Partnership programme in the UK carried out by the Department of Health, ER can be considered to consist of 16–21 different component steps. It is not known which of these component steps have the biggest impact on the individual patient with their own individual problems. It is well accepted that the ultimate success of the programme relies on adopting as many elements of the pathway and a piecemeal adoption usually results in a failure of the programme [18]. In a large prospective observational study of more than 900 colorectal patients within ER, a significant association between improved protocol adherence and post-operative outcome was demonstrated. Furthermore, patients with high compliance to ER protocol had 25% lower post-operative complication rate and 50% lower risk of post-operative symptoms delaying discharge. The study also showed a dose–response relationship between adherence to the ER protocol and improved surgical outcome. Nearly all pre-operative ER elements influenced the post-operative outcome but intravenous fluid management and pre-operative carbohydrate intake were the major independent predictors of outcome.

Massen et al. [6] conducted a multi-centre study within the ERAS group that showed a high compliance with pre-operative and operative measures but low compliance of post-operative measures. ER was established in all centres that contributed in this study, accounting for high compliance with pre- and intra-operative elements. This was reinforced by their finding that the factors most strongly associated with protocol compliance were familiarity of the patients and organisations with ER and previous exposure to fast track concepts (hazard ratio 2.28). The post-operative elements, such as early mobilisation and feeding, withdrawal of intravenous fluid and epidural analgesia had a compliance rate of only 40–50%. A similar result has also been shown in the Yeovil study, examining 385 cases who underwent laparoscopic colorectal resections within the ER programme with approximately 60% compliance of post-operative variables [19]. It could be argued that the post-operative variables of the ER are in fact an end product or the outcome of pre- and intra-operative elements of the ER pathway.

In institutions where ER is embedded in their normal practice, there must be other reasons for failure to comply with the post-operative elements. Hence, the term 'compliance' with post-operative elements of ER is rather a misnomer, and it should be addressed as a 'deviation' from the pathway.

Deviations in the Post-operative Enhanced Recovery Pathway

In the Yeovil study [19, 20], specifically addressing post-operative deviation from ER pathway, ER deviations were noted in 159 out of 385 patients (41.3%). This has resulted in prolonged LOS (more than one week) in only 90 patients (23.3%). Deviations due to continuation of intravenous fluids occurred in 117 (30.3%), epidural failure in 92 patients (24%), failure to mobilise in 65 patients (17%), development of ileus in 42 patients (11%), re-catheterise in 38 pateints (10%). On multi-variate analysis, deviation from the post-operative elements of ER appears to be the most significant in terms of association with delayed discharge. Interestingly, patient factors appear not to influence delayed discharge. Univariate analysis identified operative time > 5 hours and blood loss > 500ml as being associated with delayed discharge, but they were not significant predictors in multivariate analysis, due to the overwhelming influence of the post-operative factors [21] Also, it was noticed that failure of ER was noticed to result from several deviations of the pathway, while patients who deviated in one or two post-operative variables were still likely to be discharged within the median LOS in 80% of cases [20].

Causes of Deviation in ER

Patients who may deviate in the post-operative recovery in ER can be classified into two main categories:

1. Deviation due to surgical or medical complications
2. Deviation in patients who have no complications

1. *Deviation due to surgical complications*: Although the emphasis of ER is focused on preventing post-operative medical complication by early mobilisation, ER does not preclude surgical complications such as anastomotic dehiscence, bleeding or mechanical bowel obstruction. In fact, ER may facilitate the early detection of surgical complications by exacerbating a secondary ileus or an early obstruction in patients intolerant of early feeding. Deviation from an ER protocol can therefore be a valuable early warning sign for complications. Part of the problem, particularly with laparoscopic surgery, is that complications can present in an insidious manner and remain undiagnosed until a late stage when life-threatening sequelae such as septic shock develop. In this regard, deviation from the ER protocol at an early stage, in terms of intolerance of oral intake or unexpected poor mobility, become a very valuable early warning sign towards early detection and management of complications.

2. *Deviation in patients with no complications*: Deviation in the post-operative ER pathway in patients with no complications may present as: (1) impaired functional recovery and or (2) ileus. Both these factors are consequent to the physiological response to surgical trauma. They may also be consequent to or compounded by medical or surgical complications. Hence the diagnosis of this category should be made after excluding complications in general especially technical problems.

Prediction of Deviations in Enhanced Recovery

The concept of studying prediction of deviation in ER at the pre-operative stage is valid to allow a modified pathway be put in place for these patients. This, however, remains a challenge due to the multifactorial elements of ER.

Several predictive factors for ER deviation have been identified by uni- and multi-variate analyses including ASA III or IV, prior abdominal surgery, obesity, nutritional status, surgeon experience and case load. On analysing the intra-operative factors that predict length of post-operative stay at Yeovil, total operative time and a blood loss were significant predictors on uni-variant analysis [21].

Benign colorectal diseases (such as diverticular disease, Crohn's disease) and conversion to open and pre-operative haemoglobin level were predictors of deviation from the ER pathway and prolonged length of stay [22]. Deviation from the post-operative elements of ER appears to be the most significant in terms of association with delayed discharge [20] A score for predicting delayed discharge at 48 hours post-operatively is currently under evaluation at Yeovil.

Signs of Early Deviation from ER

If pre-operative prediction of the success or failure of ER is proven to be difficult, vigilance of the early signs and symptoms of deviation is essential. In the UK, the National Patient Safety Agency has reviewed the circumstances behind missed complications [23]. Importantly, their observations lead to the conclusion that in addition to standard post-operative monitoring and early warning scores, a patient safety checklist should occur during the second 12-h period after surgery and that this should determine the presence of the following symptoms and signs:

- Abdominal pain needing opiate analgesia
- Anorexia or reluctance to drink
- Reluctance to mobilise
- Nausea
- Vomiting
- Tachycardia
- Abdominal tenderness
- Abdominal distension
- Poor urine output
- Cardiac arrhythmia

Recognising these factors is key to identifying complications at an early stage and is a key attribute of an experienced ER team. On their own, the risk factors for ER deviation are not a reason for withdrawal from an ER pathway but need to be taken into account and consideration given to tailor the pathway to the patient.

Hence, ER deviation can represent a valuable albeit non-specific warning sign in post-operative care, providing an opportunity to detect complications or an impaired functional capacity and to take remedial action at an early stage.

Late Deviation from ER

Deviation from the ER protocol at a later stage can be an equally important indicator for intervention. If a patient fails to meet target discharge criteria, this can provide an opportunity for further review to exclude a late medical or surgical complication. The majority of such patients have made an uncomplicated recovery but due to fatigue or frailty they failed to make a full functional recovery to be discharged. In these instances, the ER team should have already planned for such an eventuality and have in place a plan and facility for ongoing care (such as a step down or rehabilitation ward). The socio-economic class may influence the level of support after discharge from hospital; hence there may be some variations in adhering to strict discharge criteria in certain parts of the country and from the UK to different European health systems.

Equally, following discharge, there should be a local protocol with criteria and a point of contact for the discharged patient to contact the ER team in the event of encountering problems. Alternatively, the ER team may choose to follow-up the discharged patient by telephone review.

Failure in Enhanced Recovery

As it has been stated earlier, deviation from the ER pathway does not necessarily mean a failure of ER and in fact it has been shown that majority of patients who deviate in one or two elements still make a good recovery and are discharge within 6 days [20].

ER failure seems to result from multiple failures in the pathway, and those patients are usually withdrawn from the ER pathway and a more tailored programme is established.

The underlying factors that may lead to ER failure will be examined in this chapter under four categories with some case scenarios in each:

1. Physiological
2. Surgical
3. Anaesthetic
4. Implementation.

Physiological Factors

Stress response to surgical trauma initiates catabolic changes with a net breakdown of glycogen, fat and protein as well as initiating neuroendocrine, immune and systemic inflammatory cascades.

A component part of the metabolic response to trauma in terms of gluconeogenesis and insulin resistance can be ameliorated by avoiding prolonged fasting and by carbohydrate pre-loading with the ER protocol. Furthermore, the neural and endocrine response to pain can be ameliorated by effective analgesia and a partial sympathetic blockade may be achieved by an epidural.

Depending on the severity of the stress response, these can be obstacles to recovery or can be beneficial to recovery. A further problem is that an exaggerated but normal physiological response following surgery can sometimes be difficult to distinguish at an early stage from that arising following a medical or surgical complication.

In a well-established ER unit, the physiological factors become the principal cause of failure in an ER protocol as the other causes are diminished. Although the main principle of ER is reducing surgical stress, in certain occasions ER fails to completely abolish the physiological response to surgical trauma. The majority of patients with reasonable functional reserve continue to cope well with the residual stress and overall succeed in ER with short length of stay. Those who lack this reserve, however usually fail ER, resulting in prolonged length of stay.

> *Case scenario 1:* An 81-year-old ASAII female undergoes elective laparoscopic high anterior resection on an ER programme. She tolerates normal diet on the first post-operative day and her pain is controlled with a thoracic epidural, paracetamol and ibuprofen analgesia. On the second post-operative day she passes flatus but experiences nausea and vomits once, but otherwise is clinically well.
>
> How should be the pathway be altered or adjusted for her?

This is an example of an early post-operative ileus, which is a common benign condition that overlaps with post-operative nausea and vomiting. It usually occurs in the first 2–3 days after bowel resection and is short-lived, lasting for 24 h or less with the patient remaining clinically well. The management here is to clinically assess the patient, exclude acute gastric dilatation, surgical and medical complications and, depending on the severity, withhold the ER for 24 h or less. The patient should be managed with the use of anti-emetics, GI tract rest and reinstate intravenous fluids if required, before reinstating oral fluids and diet when symptoms subside. A nasogastric tube is required usually only with acute gastric dilatation or continued vomiting and abdominal distension. Patients with this condition usually continue to succeed in ER.

> *Case scenario 2:* A 75-year-old ASAIII male undergoes elective laparoscopic high anterior resection. He passes flatus and tolerates diet on the first post-operative day. However, on the third post-operative day he develops nausea, distension and vomiting. A nasogastric tube is

passed and IVI started. Despite this, he has persisting and marked distension and, on the fourth post-operative day develops mild abdominal tenderness and a white cell count of 23 and CRP 272.

A CT scan suggests a distal small bowel obstruction and some free fluid in the pelvis and a rectal contrast study was inconclusive. The patient is not improving and taken to theatre. At laparotomy he has a distended non-obstructed small bowel and a distended large bowel and healthy anastomosis. He has a loop ileostomy fashioned with a flatus tube passed through the distal limb into the colon. He thereafter makes a full recovery and is discharged home on day 10.

This is an example of a prolonged post-operative ileus, which is defined as nausea, vomiting and abdominal distension that lasts or is of onset more than 3 days post-operatively. Excluding a surgical complication is essential here and thereafter the management is usually supportive – withdrawal from the ER pathway, intravenous fluids and correction of electrolyte abnormalities and nasogastric tube if vomiting. Parenteral nutrition is not usually required unless the ileus lasts more than a week or unless there is evidence pre-operatively of malnutrition. There is no evidence that prokinetics hasten the recovery from ileus [25]. In the recovery phase of ileus, double-strength dioralyte or St. Mark's solution supplemented with oral nutritional supplement can ameliorate the high-volume fluid losses that can result from enterocyte dysfunction. Although with hindsight the above case did not need a laparotomy, this was the only way to establish a definitive diagnosis. The abdominal distension meant that laparoscopy was not feasible. In the majority of cases of prolonged post-operative ileus, after exclusion of medical or surgical complication (such as early obstruction or anastomotic leak), the patient is managed conservatively but with a withdrawal from the ER and prolonged length of stay.

The incidence of prolonged post-operative ileus is decreasing with advances in anaesthetic and surgical techniques and ER. In open surgery with conventional recovery, the incidence of prolonged post-operative ileus has dropped from 40% to 50% while this has decreased significantly with the introduction of laparoscopy and ER is about 10% with laparoscopic technique and ER [26]. These effects may be further enhanced with opiate-sparing analgesic regimens, early mobilisation, prokinetics and gum chewing [24].There was a low incidence of post-operative ileus with a median time to defecation of 2 days that mirrored the median time to discharge.

Surgical Factors

Surgical performance is a critical determinant of ER's success or failure. ER cannot compensate for poor surgical performance and a high degree of suspicion is required to rule out a technical or surgical complication.

Case scenario 3: A 74-year-old ASAII male undergoes elective laparoscopic anterior resection. He goes home on day 3 tolerating normal diet and with a care package including a point of contact. On the fifth post-operative day however he feels unwell and distended, vomits and is unable to tolerate diet or fluids. He contacts the ward and is subsequently readmitted. He is distended with lower abdominal tenderness, has a high white cell count of 19 and CRP of 270. A CT shows a large presacral collection with free intraperitoneal air. At laparotomy he has an anastomotic dehiscence which is taken down and a Hartmann's procedure was performed.

ER does not have any impact in reducing surgical complications such as anastomotic dehiscence. Usually there are some indications in the early post-operative period for those patients who are likely to develop this complication, such as abdominal pain, ileus or raised inflammatory markers. In some groups of patients however, this can be very difficult especially if they are fully mobile, tolerating normal diet and passing flatus. It could be argued that patients should not be discharged following bowel surgery until they open their bowel. Conversely this may result in unnecessarily delayed discharge in the majority of patients and anastomotic dehiscence can still occur even with normal bowel function. Clearly, this patient has been discharged home having satisfied discharge criteria and with clear written instructions and a point of contact should problems arise. Some ER units have a policy of daily telephone review.

Anaesthetic Factors

Changes in anaesthetic practice, analgesia and peri-operative fluid management have all made significant contributions to ameliorating the stress of surgery and improving outcomes for the ER patient. This change in anaesthetic practice confers greater advantage to the physiologically frail patient. Similar to surgery, the anaesthetic approach can be modified according to the patient's co-morbidities and pathology.

A thorough pre-operative assessment of physiological function not only aids in tailoring this approach but can also help in setting the expectations for the patient's functional recovery and discharge planning.

> *Case scenario 4:* A 65-year-old morbid obese female underwent laparoscopic sigmoid resection for diverticular disease in a semi-elective list, which required conversion to open due to a large inflammatory mass in the sigmoid colon. Post-operatively, the patient remained drowsy for 2–3 h in recovery. After that, the patient complained of pain, the anaesthetic team was called and the epidural was increased. She now has effective epidural analgesia but with a blood pressure of 80/40 mmHg and a pulse of 90. How would you manage the patient?

The first step is clearly to exclude a surgical complication such as post-operative bleeding but this can be difficult by clinical examination alone in such instances. Epidural hypotension without tachycardia can usually be safely tolerated in the healthy patient but in the co-morbid patient may require administration of i.v. fluid. Clearly, this patient required high infusion rate of epidural to achieve optimum pain control. If hypotension persists despite fluid challenges, consider administration of vasoconstrictor such as metaraminol or ephedrine, which usually requires transfer to a high-dependency unit.

> *Case scenario 5:* A 39-year-old female with small bowel Crohn's who has been managed on a long-term analgesia undergoes laparoscopic recurrent ileocolic resection and multiple sticturoplasties. Pre-operatively the patient had patchy epidural cover and the decision was to have a buvicaine only epidural and run a morphine PCA simultaneously. What are the expectations of her recovery?

It is recognised that inflammatory bowel disease can make post-operative pain management particularly challenging as a result of pain modulation and long-term analgesic use. Sub-optimal pain control may result in poor motivation in this group of patients as well as making it harder for them to comply with other components of ER. Hence, supplementing epidural analgesia to achieve optimum pain control is necessary. This involves the multi-modal approach for analgesia including regular paracetamol, non-steroidal anti-inflammatory drugs as well as opioids. Although alternative analgesics to opiates are clearly desirable, they are not always effective. Baseline opiate analgesia (considering the previous opiate requirement) are usually insufficient in these patients and alternative analgesia, such as trans-versus abdominis plane blocks or rectus sheath infusion catheters, should have been explored.

Implementation Factors

Difficulties often arise in implementing all the elements of the ER pathway at an earlier stage of adopting ER. In well-established ER units, implementation factors can still be challenging and need to be overcome to sustain the initial success. This is mostly due to physical and economic barriers such as staff education, changes in shift patterns, the seniority of staff and skill mix and mixed specialty wards.

> *Case scenario 6:* A busy colorectal unit with a successful ER programme, due to financial constraints, ward closures and amalgamation with a neighbouring hospital, becomes a mixed specialty ward. There is then loss of staff and inability to recruit experienced nursing staff, stoma therapists and physiotherapists. Finally, the ER programme loses its facilitator. With this, the ER programme loses its ability to educate staff and is unable to reliably sustain a service at weekends and at times of staff shortage. How can this unit sustain ER?

Although clinical leadership and championship are essential elements in setting up and sustaining such a programme, clinicians are often too busy to supervise the daily tasks of ER and this role should be handed to a dedicated ER facilitator.

An ER facilitator is essential in anticipating and countering these problems as well as leading the team on a day-to-day basis. ER implementation failures, like most system failures, are often seen too late through the eyes of the medical or ward nursing staff or the bed managers. An experienced ER facilitator however, with a protected role, can recognise problems as they develop. This problem often arises when a unit with an established record of delivering ER underestimates the role of a dedicated facilitator who ensures compliance with the pathway, provides continual staff education, arranges regular meetings for the steering group and organises data collection.

Although the role of ER facilitator is essential in setting up and maintaining the ER programme, continual staff education is crucial to stain success of this programme. The main ethos of ER is the multidisciplinary team approach; this cannot be achieved by one person and if this person leaves or is not there the whole programme collapses. ER is a task shared by every member of the team who all have a responsibility to ensure its implementation.

The pathway must be embedded as the standard of care and it becomes the normal practice, with no other parallel pathways. The whole team must be clear on the method of management.

There will always be challenges and difficulties, but a strong commitment and resilience of the whole team is required to maintain their enthusiasm in the face of setbacks and to train new staff members in the ethos of ER; this can turn failure into success.

Top tips to sustain success in ER:
1. Firm foundations of the whole ER pathway without piece meal adoption
2. ER facilitator
3. Direct-line to ward for discharged patients
4. Continual data monitoring and staff education
5. Success in ER is measured by the overall impact on patient care
6. Early failure can be turned into success with early recognition and management of complications
7. Early ER deviation can represent a valuable albeit nonspecific warning sign in post-operative care
8. Failure to comply in one or two elements does not mean failure in ER; failure is usually due multiple deviations
9. Tailored ER pathway may be necessary for some patients
10. Resilience and confidence to overcome challenges

References

1. Wind J, Polle SW, Fung Kon Jin PH, Dejong CH, von Meyenfeldt MF, Ubbink DT, et al. Systematic review of enhanced recovery programmes in colonic surgery. Br J Surg. 2006; 93(7):800–9.
2. Eskicioglu C, Forbes SS, Aarts MA, Okrainec A, McLeod RS. Enhanced recovery after surgery (ERAS) programs for patients having colorectal surgery: a meta-analysis of randomized trials. J Gastrointest Surg. 2009;13(12):2321–9. Epub 2009 May 21.
3. Walter CJ, Collin J, Dumville JC, Drew PJ, Monson JR. Enhanced recovery in colorectal resections: a systematic review and meta-analysis. Colorectal Dis. 2009;11(4):344–53.
4. Varadhan KK, Neal KR, Dejong CH, Fearon KC, Ljungqvist O, Lobo DN. The enhanced recovery after surgery (ERAS) pathway for patients undergoing major elective open colorectal surgery: a meta-analysis of randomized controlled trials. Clin Nutr. 2010;29(4):434–40. Epub 2010 Jan 29.
5. Basse L, Hjort Jakobsen D, Billesbølle P, Werner M, Kehlet H. A clinical pathway to accelerate recovery after colonic resection. Ann Surg. 2000;232(1):51–7.
6. Maessen J, Dejong CH, Hausel J, Nygren J, Lassen K, Andersen J, et al. A protocol is not enough to implement an enhanced recovery programme for colorectal resection. Br J Surg. 2007;94(2):224–31.
7. Teeuwen PH, Bleichrodt RP, Strik C, Groenewoud JJ, Brinkert W, van Laarhoven CJ, et al. Enhanced recovery after surgery (ERAS) versus conventional postoperative care in colorectal surgery. J Gastrointest Surg. 2010;14(1):88–95. Epub 2009 Sep 25.
8. Khoo CK, Vickery CJ, Forsyth N, Vinall NS, Eyre-Brook IA. A prospective randomized controlled trial of multimodal perioperative management protocol in patients undergoing elective colorectal resection for cancer. Ann Surg. 2007;245(6):867–72.

9. Marret E, Remy C, Bonnet F, Postoperative Pain Forum Group. Meta-analysis of epidural analgesia versus parenteral opioid analgesia after colorectal surgery. Br J Surg. 2007;94(6): 665–73. Review.

10. Jørgensen H, Wetterslev J, Møiniche S, Dahl JB. Epidural local anaesthetics versus opioid-based analgesic regimens on postoperative gastrointestinal paralysis. PONV and pain after abdominal surgery. Cochrane Database Syst Rev. 2000;4:CD001893. Review.

11. Lobo DN, Bostock KA, Neal KR, Perkins AC, Rowlands BJ, Allison SP. Effect of salt and water balance on recovery of gastrointestinal function after elective colonic resection: a randomised controlled trial. Lancet. 2002;359(9320):1812–8.

12. Schwenk W, Haase O, Neudecker J, Muller J. Short term benefits for laparoscopic colorectal resection. Cochrane Database Syst Rev. 2005;3:CD003145.

13. Schwenk W, Böhm B, Haase O, Junghans T, Müller JM. Laparoscopic versus conventional colorectal resection: a prospective randomised study of postoperative ileus and early postoperative feeding. Langenbecks Arch Surg. 1998;383(1):49–55.

14. Raue W, Haase O, Junghans T, Scharfenberg M, Müller JM, Schwenk W. 'Fast-track' multimodal rehabilitation program improves outcome after laparoscopic sigmoidectomy: a controlled prospective evaluation. Surg Endosc. 2004;18(10):1463–8. Epub 2004 Aug 26.

15. MacKay G, Ihedioha U, McConnachie A, Serpell M, Molloy RG, O'Dwyer PJ. Laparoscopic colonic resection in fast-track patients does not enhance short-term recovery after elective surgery. Colorectal Dis. 2007;9(4):368–72.

16. Basse L, Jakobsen DH, Bardram L, Billesbølle P, Lund C, Mogensen T, et al. Functional recovery after open versus laparoscopic colonic resection: a randomized, blinded study. Ann Surg. 2005; 241(3):416–23.

17. Khan S, Wilson T, Ahmed J, Owais A, MacFie J. Quality of life and patient satisfaction with enhanced recovery protocols. Colorectal Dis. 2010;12(12):1175–82.

18. Gustafsson UO, Hausel J, Thorell A, Ljungqvist O, Soop M, Nygren J, et al. Adherence to the enhanced recovery after surgery protocol and outcomes after colorectal cancer surgery. Arch Surg. 2011;146(5):571–7.

19. Smart NJ, Brigic A, Ockrim J, Allison AS, Kennedy RH, Francis NK. Factors influencing deviation and failure from enhanced recovery protocol following laparoscopic colorectal resections: what lessons can we learn? Association of coloproctology meeting, Birmingham, 20–23 June 2011.

20. Brigic A, Smart NJ, Ockrim J, Kennedy RH, Francis NK. Deviations from enhanced recovery protocols following laparoscopic colorectal resections'. International surgical congress of association of surgeons of GB&I 2011, Bournemouth, 11–13 May 2011.

21. Boulind C, Smart N, Brigic A, Pring T, Ockrim J, Kennedy RH, Francis N. Operative factors that predict outcome in enhanced recovery after laparoscopic colorectal surgery. 19th international congress of the European association of endoscopic surgeons, Torino, 15–18 June 2011.

22. Burkill C, Boulind C, Noble H, Allison A, Ockrim J, Kennedy RH, Francis NK. Factors predict outcome in enhanced recovery programme following laparoscopic colorectal resection: multi-variant analysis. The association of surgeons of GB & I, Glasgow, May 2009.

23. Laparoscopic surgery: failure to recognise post-operative deterioration. National patient safety agency –NHS. National reporting and learning service. Central Alert System (CAS) reference: NPSA/2010/RRR016 23 September 2010 www.nrls.npsa.nhs.uk/resources.

24. Noble EJ, Harris R, Hosie KB, Thomas S, Lewis SJ. Gum chewing reduces postoperative ileus? A systematic review and meta-analysis. Int J Surg. 2009;7(2):100–5.

25. Traut U, Brügger L, Kunz R, Pauli-Magnus C, Haug K, Bucher H and Koller, MT. "Cochrane database of systematic reviews." Cochrane Database Syst Rev. 2008 Jan 23;(1):CD004930.

26. Boulind C, Yeo M, Burkill C, Witt A, James E, Ewings P, Kennedy RH, Francis N. Factors predicting deviation from an enhanced recovery programme and delayed discharge after laparoscopic colorectal surgery. Colorectal disease 2011 in press.

Chapter 11
Data Collection and Audit

Jonas O.M. Nygren and Olle Ljungqvist

There is a growing awareness worldwide that continuous quality improvements and adherence to evidence-based guidelines are of major importance in health care. However, despite universal acceptance of benefit from the measurement of quality in health care, there are currently no generally accepted standards for the benchmarking of performance and quality. The Enhanced Recovery After Surgery (ERAS) Study Group, an international working group, has developed one such system and collected a large international database [1].

Measuring standards and auditing health care quality, in itself, drives continuing improvement. In addition, publicly released performance data also improves results due to identification of the best performers and also the concern health care providers have for their public image and reputation [2].

In a recent update of a Cochrane review comprising 188 studies it was concluded that audit and feedback can be effective in improving professional practice [3]. Even though the effects are generally small to moderate, the relative effectiveness of audit and feedback is likely to be greater when adherence to recommended practice is low at the baseline, and when feedback is delivered more intensively. Two recent Cochrane Review updates showed that, in addition to regular audit, continuing educational meetings and outreach educational visits were interventions that improved professional practice and patient outcomes [4, 5]. The effects were similar to other types of continuing medical education, such as audit and feedback. Another Cochrane review concluded that printed educational materials when used alone had a beneficial effect on process outcomes (e.g. X-ray requests, smoking cessation activities, medication), but not on patient outcomes. However, the clinical

J.O.M. Nygren (✉)
Department of Surgery, Ersta Hospital and Karolinska Institutet at Danderyds Hospital,
Stockholm, Sweden

O. Ljungqvist
Department of Surgery, Örebro University Hospital, Örebro, Sweden

N. Francis et al. (eds.), *Manual of Fast Track Recovery for Colorectal Surgery*,
Enhanced Recovery, DOI 10.1007/978-0-85729-953-6_11,
© Springer-Verlag London Limited 2012

significance of the observed effect was not clear and the effectiveness of educational materials compared to other interventions was uncertain [6].

In a recent systematic review it was concluded that quality improvement strategies that were clinician/patient-driven had a stronger evidence of effectiveness than those that were manager/policy-driven [7]. There are reports from successful, complex, clinician-driven, implementation projects in health care such as the Surviving Sepsis Campaign [8]. In this study of 15,022 critically ill patients from 165 centres, substantial improvements in outcome were found when guidelines were implemented. After having established evidence-based recommendations and guidelines, compliance (a measurement of the frequency with which guidelines that are known to improve outcome were implemented) improved from 18% in the initial phase of the project, to 36% after a 2-year implementation period. Although an ambitious goal was set of reducing mortality by one-third, the improvement in compliance with treatment guidelines was associated with a significant reduction in mortality, from 37% to 30.8%.

Measurement of the compliance with which interventions that improve clinical recovery are implemented allows the use of a structured audit based on an assessment of change in compliance. This facilitates implementation of the change, providing tools for improvement in clinical care. However, when more complex clinical pathways are to be evaluated, the data collection also becomes more involved and resource demanding. This then generates more data to evaluate, increasing the number of factors in clinical practice that can influence outcome. Such complexity is particularly true in the evaluation of surgical outcomes. The surgical patient's journey along their pathway involves a series of interactions in outpatient clinics, preadmission clinics, the ward, high-dependency unit and then finally back to the ward. Multiple members of staff including clinic nurses, ward nurses, specialist nurses, junior and senior surgeons, anaesthetists, physiotherapists and many other health care workers influence outcome, administering or supervising interventions that are important. This means that a large group of personnel from different units might contribute to the data collection. The complexity of such a pathway places demands on an audit system, particularly if it is used to control day-to-day care and, more so, to manage changes in clinical practice. The process of data registration is vital in order to ensure adequate data quality. This was illustrated recently when data registration by residents was analysed, revealing highly unreliable recordings despite active training. It was concluded that a specially trained nurse coordinator was necessary in order to improve the validity of recorded data [9]. Tailored, practical adaptations to facilitate data collection are also often helpful, in particular to avoid duplicate registration of data.

In a systematic review [10], it was concluded that clinical pathways act as a powerful tool to control the quality of perioperative care and should be more widely introduced into routine practice. This was particularly important for procedures with a high volume, great complexity of treatment, or a high degree of associated morbidity and mortality. Gastrointestinal surgery is a typical example of this procedure: It is usually complex surgery with high complication rates, meeting all the above criteria. A recent paper studied the content of proposed clinical pathways in digestive surgery, analysing 13 studies, selected from 510 publications, most relating to colorectal surgery. [11] The authors reported that the majority of interventions and clinical pathways in the literature were similar to those which comprise the ERAS protocol.

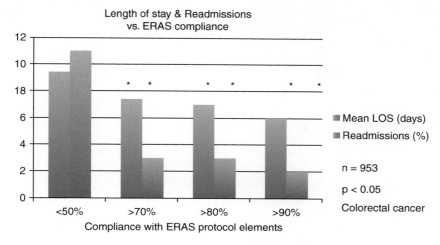

Fig. 11.1 Postoperative hospital stay (LOS) and readmission rates in patients with different compliance with ERAS protocol elements. *p<0.05 vs. low compliance (<50%) (Gustafsson et al. [14])

This protocol is a clinically derived, complex multimodal treatment protocol aiming to improve recovery and postoperative outcomes [12]. In order to successfully implement the ERAS program, a systematic process of audit has been built into the ERAS data collection system [1]. The ERAS database differs from other common audit tools in that a traditional audit system collects data on patient demographics, treatment and outcomes. What is additionally included in the ERAS system is the recording of compliance with a series of evidence-based treatment interventions that have been shown to influence outcomes. A raft of measures which provide information on different aspects of postoperative recovery, and potential factors delaying it, is incorporated into the data set to allow interrogation of the care process.

A recent study compared elective colorectal surgery patients within a clinical trial to those outside it, when both groups were treated with the same ERAS protocol [13]. The authors reported a modest improvement in compliance with ERAS interventions in the trial patients, but no or only marginal impact on postoperative outcomes such as length of stay and complications [13]. However, a larger study in 953 patients undergoing colorectal surgery demonstrated a greater improvement in compliance with pre- and perioperative ERAS components. Compliance increased from 43.3% to 70.6% during the study (2002–2004 vs. 2005–2007), which was associated with a significant reduction in symptoms delaying recovery (OR 0.53, 95% CI 0.40–0.70) and postoperative complications (OR 0.73, 95% CI 0.55–0.98) [14]. Of the 22 key ERAS variables, the use of preoperative carbohydrate loading and the restriction of perioperative intravenous fluid replacement were found to be strongly associated with improved outcomes. Across the periods, the proportion of adverse postoperative outcomes was significantly reduced with increasing adherence to the ERAS protocol (>70%, >80%, >90%) compared with low ERAS adherence (<50%) (Figs. 11.1 and 11.2).

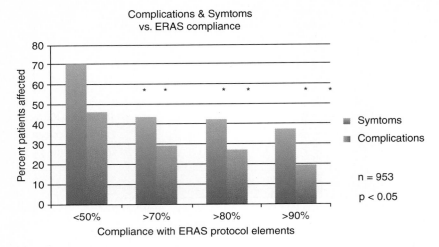

Fig. 11.2 Symtoms delaying recovery and postoperative complication rates in patients with different compliance with ERAS protocol elements. *p<0.05 vs. low compliance (<50%) (Gustafsson et al. [14])

Audit is a key instrument for clinicians aiming to implement the ERAS programme. This is the only way to gather the necessary information on compliance with the programme during the change process. By capturing details of where in the pathway there are problems, one may examine the compliance for interventions that deal with those specific issues, thus providing objectivity when problems are solved. This helps to direct future education and the modification of other interventions when necessary.

By auditing the details of the key elements of the clinical pathway it is often easier to understand the occurrence of certain complications. An example of this would be the ability to easily review the fluid balance of patients if a sudden increase in cardiac complications has been revealed, or perhaps when problems with bowel function secondary to ileus occur. Both ileus and cardiac complications may result from fluid overload and this association can be detected by using the audit. In addition to offer the local group of clinicians an improved overview of their clinical practice, the ERAS audit system also provides relevant feedback on clinical outcomes that are important for patients, health care providers and other decision makers.

References

1. Maessen J et al. A protocol is not enough to implement an enhanced recovery programme for colorectal resection. Br J Surg. 2007;34(2):224–31.
2. Mayer EK et al. Appraising the quality of care in surgery. World J Surg. 2009;33(8):1584–93.
3. Jamtvedt G et al. Audit and feedback: effects on professional practice and health care outcomes. Cochrane Database Syst Rev. 2006;2:CD000259.

4. Forsetlund L et al. Continuing education meetings and workshops: effects on professional practice and health care outcomes. Cochrane Database Syst Rev. 2009;2:CD003030.
5. O'Brien MA et al. Educational outreach visits: effects on professional practice and health care outcomes. Cochrane Database Syst Rev. 2007;4:CD000409.
6. Farmer AP et al. Printed educational materials: effects on professional practice and health care outcomes. Cochrane Database Syst Rev. 2008;3:CD004398.
7. Scott I. What are the most effective strategies for improving quality and safety of health care? Intern Med J. 2009;39(6):389–400.
8. Levy MM et al. The Surviving Sepsis Campaign: results of an international guideline-based performance improvement program targeting severe sepsis. Crit Care Med. 2010;38(2): 367–74.
9. Dindo D, Hahnloser D, Clavien PA. Quality assessment in surgery: riding a lame horse. Ann Surg. 2010;251(4):766–71.
10. Ronellenfitsch U et al. Clinical pathways in surgery: should we introduce them into clinical routine? A review article. Langenbecks Arch Surg. 2008;393(4):449–57.
11. Lemmens L et al. Clinical and organizational content of clinical pathways for digestive surgery: a systematic review. Dig Surg. 2009;26(2):91–9.
12. Lasse K et al. Consensus review of optimal perioperative care in colorectal surgery: Enhanced Recovery After Surgery (ERAS) Group recommendations. Arch Surg. 2009;144(10):961–9.
13. Ahmed J et al. Compliance with enhanced recovery programmes in elective colorectal surgery. Br J Surg. 2010;97(5):754–8.
14. Gustafsson U et al. Adherence to the enhanced recovery after surgery protocol and outcomes after colorectal cancer surgery. Arch Surg. 2011;146(5):571–7.

Index

A

Action learning process, 133
Adenosine triphosphate (ATP), 20
Anaemia, 23–25
Anaerobic threshold (AT), 20
Anaesthesia
  epidural, 42–45
  local anaesthetic blocks, 100–101
  protocols, 5
  spinal anaesthesia, 99–100
Anaesthetic approach
  anaesthetist role, 50
  CO_2 pneumoperitoneum
    cardiovascular effects, 65
    head down position, 66
    pulmonary effects, 66
    renal effects, 66
  individualised goal-directed fluid therapy
    cardiac output and oxygen
      delivery, 59–61
    controversy, 62
    fluid optimisation technique, 59, 60
    fluid shifts, 58
    goal-directed therapy, 60, 62
    individualised goal-directed
      fluids, 58
    postoperative fluids, 59
    stroke volume optimisation, 59
  laparoscopic surgery
    vs. open surgery, 63–64, 68
    physiological consequences, 65
    ventilation strategy, 67
  open surgery, 63
    vs. laparoscopic surgery, 63–64, 68
    physiological consequences,
      64–65
    ventilation strategy, 66–67

postoperative care, 67–68
pre-assessment
  cardiovascular risk reduction, 54
  functional capacity, 51
  non-cardiac surgery, cardiac risk
    index, 51–53
  peri-operative complications, 54
  pre-existing disease optimisation, 53
  surgical risk factors, 50–51
secondary complications
  postoperative chest infection
    reduction, 68–69
  venous thromboembolism risk
    reduction, 69–70
  wound infection risk reduction, 70
stress response modulation, 63
surgical preparation
  anaesthesia, 56
  anti-microbial prophylaxis, 56
  hospital admission, 55
  monitoring and vascular access, 57–58
  nasogastric tubes, GI surgery, 56
  peri-operative hypothermia
    avoidance, 57
  PONV prevention, 57
  preoperative preparation, 55
  urinary drainage, 56–57
trimodal approach, 54–55
Analgesia
  administration routes, 96
  epidural analgesia, 96–99 (see also
    Epidural analgesia)
  metabolic stress response, 42–45
  methods and regional blocks, 62–63
  open and laparoscopic surgery, 106
Angiotensin-converting enzyme (ACE)
  inhibitors, 28

N. Francis et al. (eds.), *Manual of Fast Track Recovery for Colorectal Surgery*,
Enhanced Recovery, DOI 10.1007/978-0-85729-953-6,
© Springer-Verlag London Limited 2012

Angiotensin II (ATII) receptor antagonists, 28
Anti-microbial prophylaxis, 56

B
Beta blockers, 54

C
Cardiopulmonary exercise testing
        (CPET), 20, 21
Cardiovascular risk assessment
    aerobic capacity, 20
    clinical risk indices, 18–19
    functional capacity, 19–20
    12 Lead Resting ECG, 21
    non-invasive stress testing, 21, 23
    patient history and physical
            examination, 18
    perioperative mortality, 20–21
    risk evaluation and management, 21, 22
Chronic obstructive pulmonary disease
        (COPD), 23
Cyclooxygenase (COX) type 2 inhibitors, 103

D
Diabetes, 28–29
Dobutamine stress echocardiograpy (DSE), 21
Doppler-guided fluid management, 82

E
Elective abdominal surgery failure, 1
Enhanced recovery after surgery (ERAS)
    anaesthetic approach (*see* Anaesthetic
            approach)
    anaesthetic protocols, 5
    auditing, 174
    barriers and troubleshooting
        finances and logistical support
                restrictions, 140
        inadequate staff numbers, 140–141
        organisational barriers, 141
        professional context, 140
        social barriers, 139–140
        time pressures and time lack, 140
    benefits, 121
    care pathway creation, 136
    change management principle
        action learning process, 133
        plan-do-study-act cycle, 132
        transformation strategy, 132–133
    clinical outcomes and monitoring,
            9–10, 136–137

colorectal surgery, 115–116
    abdominal and pelvic drainage
            avoidance, 119
    anastomotic leak avoidance, 119
    bladder catheter removal, 119–120
    epidural analgesia, 116–117
    goal-directed perioperative fluid
            administration, 115–116
    high perioperative oxygen
            concentration, 116
    laparoscopic surgery, 118
    mechanical bowel preparation, 112–113
    nasogastric tubes avoidance, 119
    normothermia maintenance, 116
    patient positioning, 117–118
    postoperative laxatives, 119
    rectal cancer recovery, 120
    single-port surgery, 120–121
    stoma training, 113, 115
    transverse incision, 118
complications
    anastomotic leak, 122–123
    nausea and vomiting, 121–122
    postoperative ileus, 122
cost savings, 135–136
data collection
    Cochrane Review updates, 171–172
    complexity, 172
    compliance, 172–174
    data registration, 172
    perioperative care quality, 172
    quality improvement strategies, 172
early mobilisation, 7–8
early oral intake promotion, 7
metabolic conditioning, 4–5
metabolic stress response
        (*see* Metabolic stress response)
multidisciplinary team members, 4
multimodal pain relief, 6–7
pain control (*see* Pain control)
patient discharge criteria, 8
perioperative fluid management
        (*see* Intravenous fluid therapy)
preadmission information
        and counselling, 4
preoperative fasting, 4
principles, 2–3
quality improvements, 135–136
staff education, 137–139
steering group
    aims of, 134
    ER facilitator, 134
    members, 133–134
    quality improvements, 135–136
    sub-groups and reports, 134

success and failure assessment, 159
　　anaesthetic factors, 167–168
　　clinical outcome measures, 160
　　compliance, 161–162
　　functional recovery, 160–161
　　implementation factors, 168–169
　　patient satisfaction, 161
　　physiological factors, 165–166
　　post-operative recovery deviations,
　　　162–164
　　surgical factors, 166–167
　surgical incisions, 6
　surgical technique, 5–6
Enhanced recovery facilitator
　care management
　　outpatient clinic, 146–147
　　postoperative recovery, 149,
　　　156–157
　　preadmission clinic, 147
　　recovery, 148–149
　　surgery, 148, 155
　　surgery admission day, 148, 155
　data collection, 149–150
　duties and responsibilities
　　clinical practice and practice
　　　development, 151
　　financial responsibility, 153
　　professional/education and training
　　　role, 152–153
　　research and audit, 152
　　risk management, 153
　　service development and management,
　　　152
　emergency and assessment ward triage
　　area, 146
　ER phone management, 145–146
　ER Programme evaluation, 150
　ER team meetings, 145
　job description, 150–151
　patient discharge information, 145
　patient documentation creation, 145
　person specification form, 153–154
　primary care, 146
　responsibilities, 143–144
Epidural anaesthesia
　metabolic stress response, 42–45
　oliguria, 87
　pain control, 97
Epidural analgesia, 5
　clinical outcomes, 160
　colorectal surgery, 96–99, 116–117
　vs. intravenous opioid analgesia, 7
　low molecular weight heparin, 70
　mid-thoracic, 85
　open surgery pulmonary function, 69

side effetcs, 96, 97
urinary catheters removal, 120
urinary retention, 56
Erythropoietin-stimulating agents (ESAs), 25

F
Fluid therapy
　cardiovascular monitoring, 80–81
　colorectal cancer, 77
　ERAS protocol
　　intraoperative, 85–86
　　postoperative, 85–86
　　preoperative, 83–85
　goal-directed therapy
　　vs. inotrope use, 82
　　oesophageal Doppler-guided fluid
　　　management, 82
　　principle, 81
　　stroke volume, 82
　restrictive/standard/liberal regimens, 78–80

H
Hyperglycaemia, 28, 38, 39, 43
Hypertension, 27–28
Hyponatraemia, 77, 78
Hypotension
　angiotensin-converting enzyme, 28
　angiotensin II receptor antagonist, 28
　epidural analgesia, 97–98
　oliguria, 86
Hypothermia
　anaesthetic contributions, 57
　colorectal surgery, 116
　fluid management, 75

I
Individualised goal-directed fluid therapy
　anaesthetic approach
　　cardiac output and oxygen delivery,
　　　59–61
　　controversy, 62
　　fluid optimisation technique, 59, 60
　　fluid shifts, 58
　　goal-directed therapy, 60, 62
　　individualised goal-directed fluids, 58
　　postoperative fluids, 59
　　stroke volume optimisation, 59
　　vs. inotrope use, 82
　　oesophageal Doppler-guided fluid
　　　management, 82
　　perioperative fluid administration,
　　　115–116

Individualised goal-directed fluid therapy (cont.)
    principle, 81
    stroke volume, 82
Intravenous fluid therapy
    fluid therapy (see Fluid therapy)
    fluid types, 77
    inappropriate fluid balance
        balanced salt solutions, 76
        cellular level saline, 76
        fluid restriction, 76
        salt and water fluctuations, 75
        sodium and water requirements, 74
        sodium chloride, 74–75
        third-space losses, 74

K
Ketamine, 104–105

L
Laparoscopic resection, 5
Lee index, 18
LiDCO system, 81
Low molecular weight heparin (LMWH), 70

M
Magnesium, 105
Metabolic equivalent of task (MET), 19
Metabolic stress response
    bowel preparation, 41, 44
    cancer, 40
    carbohydrate treatment, 44
    diabetes, 40
    epidural anaesthesia and analgesia, 42–45
    injury, 37–38
    insulin resistance and complications
        glucose uptake, 38
        hyperglycaemia, 38
        postoperative metabolism, 39
        protein balance, 39
        stress-induced insulin resistance, 39
        surgical stress and fatigue, 38–39
        tissue healing, 39
    malnourished patient, 40
    postoperative oral intake, 45
    preoperative fasting, 41–42, 44
    preoperative nutritional support, 40–41
    preoperative outpatient visit, 43–44
Morphine, 95
Multidisciplinary team members, 4
Multimodal pain relief, 6–7

N
National Institute for Health and Clinical
        Excellence (NICE), 25
Non-steroidal Anti-inflammatory Drugs
        (NSAIDS), 7, 103
Nutritional Risk Score (NRS), 26

O
Obesity, 27
Opioids, 95
    strong opioids, 101–102
    weaker opioids, 102–103

P
Pain control
    anaesthesia (see Anaesthesia)
    analgesia (see Analgesia)
    beta-blocker, 105
    COX–2 inhibitor, 103
    glucocorticoids, 105
    ketamine, 104–105
    lidocaine infusions, 104
    magnesium, 105
    NSAIDS, 103
    paracetamol, 103–104
    practical approach, 106
    pregabalin, 105
Paracetamol, 103–104
Patient discharge criteria, 8
Patient Education and Conditioning
        of Expectations, 30–32
Perioperative fluid management.
        See Intravenous fluid therapy
Plan-do-study-act (PDSA) cycle, 132
Postoperative nausea and vomiting (PONV)
    anaesthetic contributions, 57
    ketamine, 104
    perioperative fluid management, 86
Preadmission information
        and counselling, 4
Pre-assessment, 15
    anaemia, 23–25
    cardiovascular risk
        abdominal surgery, 17
        adverse events, 17
        aerobic capacity, 20
        clinical risk indices, 18–19
        functional capacity, 19–20
        incidence, 17
        laparoscopy, 18
        12 Lead Resting ECG, 21

non-invasive stress testing, 21, 23
patient history and physical
    examination, 18
perioperative mortality, 20–21
risk evaluation and management,
    21, 22
risk factors, 18
diabetes, 28–29
hypertension, 27–28
nutrition, 25–27
obesity, 27
pre-assessment clinics, 16
pulmonary risk, 23
smoking and high alcohol, 29
Pregabalin, 105
Pulmonary risk, 23

S
Spinal anaesthesia, 99–100
Statins, 54
Stress-induced insulin resistance, 39
Surgical incisions, 6

T
Traditional peri-operative care, 1
Transoesophageal Doppler (TOD) probes, 81
Transversus abdominis plane (TAP) block,
    100–101

V
Venous thromboembolism (VTE), 69–70

Printed by Printforce, the Netherlands